Pull Out
Code Quick Reference

ADA American Dental Association®

America's leading advocate for oral health

D4249 clinical crown lengthening – hard tissue

D4910 periodontal maintenance

VI. Prosthodontics, removable

D5110 complete denture – maxillary
D5120 complete denture – mandibular
D5130 immediate denture – maxillary
D5140 immediate denture – mandibular
D5211 maxillary partial denture – resin base (including any conventional clasps, rests and teeth)
D5212 mandibular partial denture – resin base (including any conventional clasps, rests and teeth)
D5213 maxillary partial denture – cast metal framework with resin denture bases (including any conventional clasps, rests and teeth)
D5214 mandibular partial denture – cast metal framework with resin denture bases (including any conventional clasps, rests and teeth)
D5225 maxillary partial denture – flexible base (including any clasps, rests and teeth)
D5226 mandibular partial denture – flexible base (including any clasps, rests and teeth)
D5410 adjust complete denture – maxillary

D5411 adjust complete denture – mandibular
D5421 adjust partial denture – maxillary
D5422 adjust partial denture – mandibular
D5510 repair broken complete denture base
D5520 replace missing or broken teeth – complete denture (each tooth)
D5610 repair resin denture base
D5630 repair or replace broken clasp
D5640 replace broken teeth – per tooth
D5650 add tooth to existing partial denture
D5660 add clasp to existing partial denture
D5730 reline complete maxillary denture (chairside)
D5731 reline complete mandibular denture (chairside)
D5740 reline maxillary partial denture (chairside)
D5741 reline mandibular partial denture (chairside)
D5750 reline complete maxillary denture (laboratory)
D5751 reline complete mandibular denture (laboratory)
D5820 interim partial denture (maxillary)

VII. Maxillofacial Prosthetics

D5993 maintenance and cleaning of a maxillofacial prosthesis (extra or intraoral) other than required adjustment, by report

VIII. Implant Services

D6010 surgical placement of implant body: endosteal implant
D6012 surgical placement of interim implant body for transitional prosthesis: endosteal implant
D6053 implant/abutment supported removable denture for completely edentulous arch
D6055 connecting bar – implant supported or abutment supported
D6056 prefabricated abutment – includes placement
D6057 custom abutment – includes placement
D6059 abutment supported porcelain fused to metal crown (high noble metal)
D6069 abutment supported retainer for porcelain fused to metal FPD (high noble metal)
D6092 recement implant/abutment supported crown
D6093 recement implant/abutment supported fixed partial denture

D6200 – D6999 IX. Prosthodontics, fixed

D6205	pontic – indirect resin based composite
D6210	pontic – cast high noble metal
D6240	pontic – porcelain fused to high noble metal
D6241	pontic – porcelain fused to predominantly base metal
D6242	pontic – porcelain fused to noble metal
D6245	pontic – porcelain/ceramic
D6710	crown – indirect resin based composite
D6740	crown – porcelain/ceramic
D6750	crown – porcelain fused to high noble metal
D6751	crown – porcelain fused to predominantly base metal
D6752	crown – porcelain fused to noble metal
D6790	crown – full cast high noble metal
D6930	recement fixed partial denture
D6980	fixed partial denture repair, by report

D7000 – D7999 X. Oral and Maxillofacial Surgery

D7111	coronal remnants – deciduous tooth
D7140	extraction, erupted tooth or exposed root (elevation and/or forceps removal)
D7210	surgical removal of erupted tooth requiring removal of bone and/or sectioning of tooth, and including elevation of mucoperiosteal flap if indicated
D7220	removal of impacted tooth – soft tissue
D7230	removal of impacted tooth – partially bony
D7250	surgical removal of residual tooth roots (cutting procedure)
D7286	biopsy of oral tissue – soft
D7287	exfoliative cytological sample collection
D7288	brush biopsy – transepithelial sample collection
D7311	alveoloplasty in conjunction with extractions – one to three teeth or tooth spaces per quadrant
D7510	incision and drainage of abscess – intraoral soft tissue
D7951	sinus augmentation with bone or bone substitutes
D7953	bone replacement graft for ridge preservation – per site

D8000 – D8999 XI. Orthodontics

D8080	comprehensive orthodontic treatment of the adolescent dentition
D8090	comprehensive orthodontic treatment of the adult dentition
D8670	periodic orthodontic treatment visit (as part of contract)
D8692	replacement of lost or broken retainer

D9000 – D9999 XII. Adjunctive General Services

D9110	palliative (emergency) treatment of dental pain – minor procedure
D9120	fixed partial denture sectioning
D9215	local anesthesia in conjunction with operative or surgical procedures
D9230	inhalation of nitrous oxide/anxiolysis, analgesia
D9248	non-intravenous conscious sedation
D9310	consultation – (diagnostic service provided by dentist or physician other than requesting dentist or physician
D9430	office visit for observation (regular hours)
D9630	other drugs and/or medicaments, by report (dispensed in office)
D9910	application of desensitizing medicament
D9911	application of desensitizing resin for cervical and/or root surface
D9920	behavior management, by report
D9940	occlusal guard, by report
D9951	occlusal adjustment – limited
D9972	external bleaching – per arch

Code Quick Reference

D0100 – D0999   I. Diagnostic

D0120	periodic oral evaluation
D0140	limited oral evaluation – problem focused
D0145	oral evaluation for patient under three years of age and counseling with primary caregiver
D0150	comprehensive oral evaluation – new or established patient
D0160	detailed and extensive oral evaluation – problem focused, by report
D0170	re-evaluation – limited, problem focused (established patient; not post-operative visit)
D0180	comprehensive periodontal evaluation – new or established patient
D0210	intraoral – complete series (including bitewings)
D0220	intraoral – periapical first film
D0230	intraoral – periapical each additional film
D0240	intraoral – occlusal film
D0270	bitewing – single film
D0272	bitewings – two films
D0273	bitewings – three films
D0274	bitewings – four films
D0277	vertical bitewings – 7 to 8 films
D0330	panoramic film
D0460	pulp vitality tests
D0470	diagnostic casts

D1000 – D1999   II. Preventive

D1110	prophylaxis – adult
D1120	prophylaxis – child
D1203	topical application of fluoride – child
D1204	topical application of fluoride – adult
D1206	topical fluoride varnish; therapeutic application for moderate to high risk caries patients
D1330	oral hygiene instructions
D1351	sealant – per tooth
D1352	preventive resin restoration in a moderate to high caries risk patient – permanent tooth
D1510	space maintainer – fixed – unilateral
D1515	space maintainer – fixed – bilateral
D1555	removal of fixed space maintainer

D2000 – D2999   III. Restorative

D2140	amalgam – one surface, primary or permanent
D2150	amalgam – two surfaces, primary or permanent
D2160	amalgam – three surfaces, primary or permanent
D2161	amalgam – four or more surfaces, primary or permanent
D2330	resin-based composite – one surface, anterior
D2750	crown – porcelain fused to high noble metal
D2751	crown – porcelain fused to predominantly base metal
D2752	crown – porcelain fused to noble metal
D2783	crown – 3/4 porcelain/ceramic
D2790	crown – full cast high noble metal

D2331 resin-based composite – two surfaces, anterior
D2332 resin-based composite – three surfaces, anterior
D2335 resin-based composite – four or more surfaces or involving incisal angle (anterior)
D2390 resin-based composite crown, anterior
D2391 resin-based composite – one surface, posterior
D2392 resin-based composite – two surfaces, posterior
D2393 resin-based composite – three surfaces, posterior
D2394 resin-based composite – four surfaces, posterior
D2643 onlay – porcelain/ceramic – three surfaces
D2644 onlay – porcelain/ceramic – four or more surfaces
D2710 crown – resin (indirect)
D2740 crown – porcelain/ceramic substrate

D2792 crown – full cast noble metal
D2920 recement crown
D2930 prefabricated stainless steel crown – primary tooth
D2940 protective restoration
D2950 core buildup, including any pins
D2951 pin retention – per tooth
D2952 cast post and core in addition to crown
D2954 prefabricated post and core in addition to crown
D2962 labial veneer (porcelain laminate) – laboratory
D2970 temporary crown (fractured tooth)
D2971 additional procedures to construct a new crown under existing partial denture framework
D2980 crown repair, by report

D3000 – D3999   IV. Endodontics

D3110 pulp cap - direct (excluding final restoration)
D3120 pulp cap - indirect (excluding final restoration)
D3220 therapeutic pulpotomy (excluding final restoration) - removal of pulp coronal to the dentinocemental junction and application of medicament
D3221 pulpal debridement, primary and permanent teeth
D3230 pulpal therapy (resorbable filling) - anterior, primary tooth (excluding final restoration)

D3310 endodontic therapy, anterior tooth (excluding final restoration)
D3320 endodontic therapy, bicuspid tooth (excluding final restoration)
D3330 endodontic therapy, molar (excluding final restoration)
D3332 incomplete endodontic therapy; inoperable or fractured tooth
D3346 retreatment of previous root canal therapy - anterior
D3347 retreatment of previous root canal therapy - bicuspid
D3348 retreatment of previous root canal therapy - molar

D4000 – D4999   V. Periodontics

D4210 gingivectomy or gingivoplasty - four or more contiguous teeth or tooth bounded spaces per quadrant
D4211 gingivectomy or gingivoplasty - one to three contiguous teeth or tooth bounded spaces per quadrant
D4230 anatomical crown exposure - four or more teeth per quadrant
D4231 anatomical crown exposure - one to three teeth per quadrant
D4240 gingival flap procedure, including root planing - four or more contiguous teeth or tooth bounded spaces per quadrant
D4241 gingival flap procedure, including root planing - one to three

D4260 osseous surgery (including flap entry and closure) - four or more contiguous teeth or tooth bounded spaces per quadrant
D4261 osseous surgery (including flap entry and closure) - one to three contiguous teeth or tooth bounded spaces per quadrant
D4263 bone replacement graft - first site in quadrant
D4271 free soft tissue graft procedure (including donor site surgery)
D4341 periodontal scaling and root planing - four or more teeth per quadrant
D4342 periodontal scaling and root planing - one to three teeth per quadrant
D4355 full mouth debridement to enable comprehensive evaluation

PRACTICAL GUIDE SERIES

CDT Companion

The ADA Practical Guide to
Dental Coding

- Dental/Medical Procedure Cross Coding

- Fold-Out CDT Quick Reference

- Clinical Coding Exercises and Scenarios

ADA American Dental Association®
America's leading advocate for oral health

Acknowledgements

This book is a result of the efforts of many dedicated individuals who participate in the development and maintenance of the CDT manual, the *Code on Dental Procedures and Nomenclature*, the ADA Dental Claim Form, and in the resolution of dental benefits related issues.

We also want to acknowledge the permissions to reprint:

- Artwork provided by Zimmer Dental used in the discussion of Implant procedures. These images are identified by the caption: "Image courtesy of Zimmer Dental."

- Artwork provided by Imaging Sciences International, Inc. used in the Coding Exercises section. These images are identified by the caption: "Image courtesy of Imaging Sciences International, Inc. www.i-cat.com"

The CDT Companion:
Your Guide to Dental Coding

Table of Contents

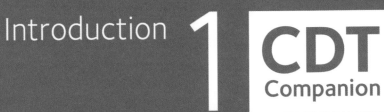

Introduction 1 CDT Companion

Chapter 1
Introduction

This book is intended as a companion to *Current Dental Terminology, CDT 2011/2012* (CDT), which contains the *Code on Dental Procedures and Nomenclature (Code)*. It is also a supplement to the ADA Continuing Education and Lifelong Learning (CELL) workshop, *The Code: Your Gateway to Accuracy*. Whether you are a general dentist, specialty dentist, dental hygienist, dental assistant or office manager, this book will help you develop and refine your knowledge and understanding of the current dental codes and your coding skills so that you can prepare dental claims more effectively.

This book will help you:

- Learn the *Code's* history and how to recommend changes

- Understand major *Code* changes that are effective as of January 1, 2011

- Give you an opportunity to apply the *Code* through clinical situations

- Cross reference dental procedure codes to medical procedure codes when preparing claims against a patient's medical benefit plan

The *Code on Dental Procedures and Nomenclature* as published in the CDT manual is like other code sets because it provides standardized information and creates a common platform of understanding. The *Code* is also the named HIPAA national standard to document dental procedures, and to communicate accurate information on procedures and services to agencies involved in adjudicating dental claims. Dentist-Payer communication is increasingly electronic, which requires the use of standard codified information. Although the *Code's* use in insurance claims remains important, other uses are gaining in significance.

Information age technologies require the use of standardized codes for effective Internet and other electronic communications. Practice management software is already procedure code driven. In addition, government, patients and health care professionals have increasing interest in standard electronic health records.

In many ways the *Code* has become the vocabulary that the profession uses to describe what it does. Professional communications increasingly rely on the *Code's* nomenclatures and descriptors for precision and accuracy. Peer review and regulatory agencies consider the *Code* as an implicit description of procedures performed by practitioners.

A Brief History

The *Code* was first published in 1969 as the "Uniform Code on Dental Procedures and Nomenclature" in the *Journal of the American Dental Association* and consisted of numbers and a brief name, or nomenclature. Since 1990, the *Code* has been published in the American Dental Association's dental reference manual titled *Current Dental Terminology* (CDT). The version of the *Code* published in *CDT-1* (1990) was marked by the addition of descriptors (a written narrative that provides further definition and the intended use of a dental procedure code) for most of the procedure codes.

The American Dental Association is the copyright owner and publisher of the CDT manual and the *Code*. The *Code* is maintained by the Code Revision Committee (CRC) with new versions every two years. These revisions to the *Code* are published in the CDT manual and effective biennially, starting January 1st of every odd-numbered year. In addition to the *Code* itself, each new edition of the CDT manual includes a Q & A section; detailed claim form instructions; information on tooth numbering systems; an updated glossary; plus both alpha and numeric indexes.

The 15th version of the Code (published in CDT 2011/2012) is effective for two years, from January 1, 2011 through December 31, 2012.

Federal regulations and legislation arising from the Health Insurance Portability and Accountability Act of 1996 (HIPAA) required all payers to accept HIPAA standard electronic transactions (including the dental claim) no later than October 16, 2003. One data element on the electronic dental claim format is the dental procedure code, which must be from the *Code on Dental Procedures and Nomenclature* – specifically the version of the *Code* that is effective on the date of service.

The *Code's* Purpose

The *Code* supports three broad categories of activities:

- Treatment planning and clinical record keeping
- Claims submission and encounter reporting
- Professional communication and education

The *Code* provides uniformity, consistency and specificity in documenting dental treatment. It also supports recording of patient services rendered and facilitates claims administration.

Treatment plans must be developed according to professional standards, *not* according to provisions of the dental benefit contract. Always keep in mind that the existence of a procedure code does not guarantee that the procedure is a covered service.

The *Code's* Organization and Structure

2

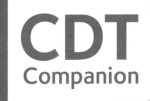

Chapter 2
The *Code's* Organization and Structure

Categories of Service

The *Code* is organized into twelve categories of service, each with its own series of five-digit alphanumeric codes. These categories reflect dental services that are considered similar in purpose.

#	Name	Code Range	Description in commonly used terms*
I.	Diagnostic	D0100–D0999	Examinations, X-rays, pathology lab procedures
II.	Preventive	D1000–D1999	Cleanings (prophy), fluoride, sealants
III.	Restorative	D2000–D2999	Fillings, crowns and other related procedures
IV.	Endodontics	D3000–D3999	Root canals
V.	Periodontics	D4000–D4999	Surgical and non-surgical treatments of the gums and tooth supporting bone
VI.	Prosthodontics – removable	D5000–D5899	Dentures – partials and "flippers"
VII.	Maxillofacial Prosthetics	D5900–D5999	Facial, ocular and various other prostheses.
VIII.	Implant Services	D6000–D6199	Implants and implant restorations
IX.	Prosthodontics – fixed	D6200–D6999	Cemented bridges
X.	Oral & Maxillofacial Surgery	D7000–D7999	Extractions, surgical procedures, biopsies, treatment of fractures and injuries
XI.	Orthodontics	D8000–D8999	Braces
XII.	Adjunctive General Services	D9000–D9999	Miscellaneous services including anesthesia, professional visits, therapeutic drugs, bleaching, occlusal adjustment, mouthguards

* The language used in the "Description..." column is not technical terminology. It has been simplified using common non-clinical terms.

Subcategories

Within most categories of service the *Code* is further subdivided into subcategories. For example, the Diagnostic category is subdivided as follows:

I. Diagnostic
- Clinical Oral Evaluations
- Radiographs/Diagnostic Imaging
- Tests and Examinations
- Oral Pathology Laboratory

All categories of service have their codes grouped within subcategories to facilitate navigation through the *Code*. There is only one exception; there are no subcategories within Maxillofacial Prosthetics.

Some subcategories are further divided for even more precision, for example, the Implant Services category has four subcategories. The implant supported prosthetics subcategory is further subdivided into seven sub-subcategories, as follows:

VIII. Implant Services
- Pre-surgical Services
- Surgical Services
- Implant Supported Prosthetics
    - Supporting Structures
    - Implant/Abutment Supported Removable Dentures
    - Implant /Abutment Supported Fixed Dentures (Hybrid Prosthesis)
    - Single Crowns, Abutment Supported
    - Single Crowns, Implant Supported
    - Fixed Partial Denture, Abutment Supported
    - Fixed Partial Denture, Implant Supported
- Other Implant Services

It should be noted that some of the codes are not in numerical order within these subcategories.

Components of a Dental Procedure Code

Every dental procedure code within a Category of Service of the *Code on Dental Procedures and Nomenclature* has at least the first two and sometimes all three of the following components:

Procedure Code – A five-character alphanumeric code beginning with the letter "D" that identifies a specific dental procedure. Each Procedure Code is printed in **boldface** type in the CDT manual and cannot be changed or abbreviated. As of January 1, 2000 the letter "D" replaced the numeral "0" as the first character of a dental procedure code. The ADA made this change to enable the *Code* to be named as the HIPAA standard for reporting dental procedures, and to differentiate dental procedure codes from the American Medical Association CPT-4® anesthesia codes.

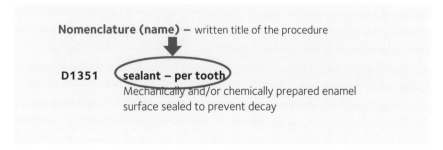

Dental Procedure Code – five character alphanumeric beginning with "D"

D1351   **sealant – per tooth**
Mechanically and/or chemically prepared enamel
surface sealed to prevent decay

Nomenclature – The written, literal definition of a Procedure Code. Each code has Nomenclature that is printed in **boldface** type in the CDT manual. Nomenclature may be abbreviated only when printed on claim forms or other documents that are subject to space limitation. Any such abbreviation does not constitute a change to the Nomenclature.

Nomenclature (name) – written title of the procedure

D1351   **sealant – per tooth**
Mechanically and/or chemically prepared enamel
surface sealed to prevent decay

Descriptor – A written narrative that provides further definition and the intended use of a dental procedure code. A Descriptor is not provided for every procedure code. Descriptors that apply to a series of procedure codes may precede that series of codes; otherwise a descriptor will follow the applicable procedure code and its nomenclature. When present, descriptors are printed in regular typeface in the CDT manual. Descriptors cannot be added, abbreviated or otherwise changed.

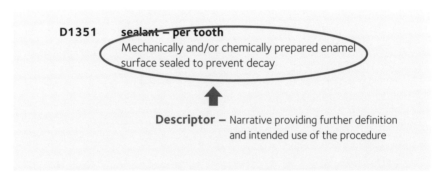

D1351   sealant – per tooth
         Mechanically and/or chemically prepared enamel
         surface sealed to prevent decay

Descriptor – Narrative providing further definition
and intended use of the procedure

Descriptors are a very important component. Knowing what is within a descriptor can help determine whether the procedure code is correct for the service being provided to a patient. This information can also help resolve questions about the accuracy of claim submissions.

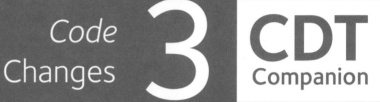

Code
Changes **3** **CDT**
Companion

ADA American Dental Association®
America's leading advocate for oral health

Chapter 3
Code Changes

Effective January 1, 2011

There are two symbols used in the CDT manual, one to identify an addition to the *Code*, and another to identify a revision.

- ● **Additions**
- ▲ **Revisions**

There is no symbol for a deletion. In the CDT manual any deleted procedure codes are noted in the "Changes..." chapter and in the "Numeric Index."

There were 118 code change requests received in the revision cycle that led to the version of the Code published in *CDT 2011/2012*. Every request was considered by each member of the CRC. Out of all the requests, 8 additions (new codes) and 19 revisions (18 to existing code nomenclatures or descriptors, and 1 to a subcategory of service in endodontics) were accepted; no codes were deleted.

A summary of *Code* additions and revisions that are effective January 1, 2011 follows.

Category of Service	New	Revised	Deleted
Diagnostics	None	▲ D0486	None
Preventive	● D1352	None	None
Restorative	None	▲ D2940	None
Endodontics	● D3354	▲ D3351 ▲ D3352 "Apexification / Recalcification..." subcategory	None
Periodontics	None	▲ D4263 ▲ D4264 ▲ D4266 ▲ D4267 ▲ D4320 ▲ D4321	None
Removable Prosthodontics	None		
Maxillofacial Prosthetics	● D5992 ● D5993	None	None
Implant Services	None	▲ D6055	None
Fixed Prosthodontics	● D6254 ● D6795	▲ D6950	None
Oral & Maxillofacial Surgery	● D7251 ● D7295	▲ D7210 ▲ D7953 ▲ D7960	None
Orthodontics	None		
Adjunctive General Services	None	▲ D9215 ▲ D9230 ▲ D9240	None

Past Significant Changes

Council on Dental Benefit Program staff continues to receive calls from dental offices regarding these past changes.

Diagnostic

Codes 00110 (initial exam) and 00130 (emergency exam) have not been part of the *Code* since January 1, 1995.

- Several different codes might be used for an initial encounter with a patient, depending on the age or emphasis (**D0145, D0150,** and **D0180**). All of these codes have a broad scope and can be used for both new and existing patients.

- Likewise, several codes may be used to describe an evaluation related to more limited diagnostic visit which would include dental emergencies (**D0140, D0160,** and **D0170**). These codes are differentiated by the depth and extent of the "problem focused" evaluation and may be used even when the situation would not be considered an emergency.

- There are seven oral evaluation codes that recognize the cognitive skills needed for an evaluation. The descriptor of each code should be reviewed when a decision is made to report an evaluation code. For example, note the descriptor differences of the following two codes:

D0140 **limited oral evaluation – problem focused**

An evaluation limited to a specific oral health problem or complaint. This may require interpretation of information acquired through additional diagnostic procedures. Report additional diagnostic procedures separately. Definitive procedures may be required on the same date as the evaluation.

Typically, patients receiving this type of evaluation present with a specific problem and/or dental emergencies, trauma, acute infections, etc.

D0160 **detailed and extensive oral evaluation – problem focused, by report**

A detailed and extensive problem focused evaluation entails extensive diagnostic and cognitive modalities based on the findings of a comprehensive oral evaluation. Integration of more extensive diagnostic modalities to develop a treatment plan for a specific problem is required. The condition requiring this type of evaluation should be described and documented.

Examples of conditions requiring this type of evaluation may include dentofacial anomalies, complicated perio-prosthetic conditions, complex temporomandibular dysfunction, facial pain of unknown origin, conditions requiring multi-disciplinary consultation, etc.

Endodontics

Prior to the version of the *Code* published in *CDT-1* (1990), endodontic therapy was reported by the number of canals treated, with procedure codes for teeth with one, two, three or four canals. Beginning in 1990 the nomenclature of these procedure codes was changed to indicate the anatomic type of tooth. At the same time the four canal procedure code was deleted.

Report procedures by type of tooth, not by number of canals.

> **D3310**   **endodontic therapy, anterior tooth (excluding final restoration)**
>
> **D3320**   **endodontic therapy, bicuspid tooth (excluding final restoration)**
>
> **D3330**   **endodontic therapy, molar (excluding final restoration)**

Oral & Maxillofacial Surgery

Prior to January 1, 2003 there were codes for extraction of "each additional tooth" as well as "root removal." Effective January 1, 2003 these codes, **D7110, D7120** and **D7130,** were deleted and replaced by codes that placed emphasis on the extraction procedure.

- **D7140** added as a replacement for all three of the deleted codes. This code is reported for the first extraction, each additional extraction and extraction of exposed roots.

- **D7111** was added, to report extraction of a coronal remnant of primary tooth

Implant Services – An In-Depth Look

4

CDT
Companion

Chapter 4
Implant Services – An In-Depth Look

The implant category of service is somewhat unique from other categories because it includes separate procedure codes for surgical placement, for placement of the intermediary components and for the supported prosthetics. These procedure codes recognize the integrated techniques and components that allow the implant-related prosthetics to restore form and function. Once the terms in the Implant Services category are understood, it will become less challenging and even easy to document the procedures performed.

Key Terms and Concepts

Abutment: The intermediary component placed on the implant body that is used to support a prosthesis. One way implant prosthetics are differentiated is based on whether abutments are used.

> *Note:* As of January 1, 2000 the term "abutment" is only included in the nomenclatures of Implant Services procedures. Prior to January 1, 1995 the term "abutment" was used to describe a supporting (anchor) tooth in a fixed bridge. The term "retainer" is now used in lieu of "abutment" for procedures in fixed prosthodontics.

Abutment Supported Prosthesis: The final prosthetic device that is attached to the abutment, not directly to the implant body.

Implant Supported Prosthesis: The final prosthetic device that is attached directly to the implant body (there is no intermediary abutment).

Implant/Abutment Supported Prothesis: The final prosthetic device is retained, supported or stabilized by an implant body or by an intermediary abutment; there is not a direct correlation between specific teeth and the implants that support them.

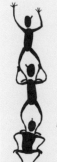
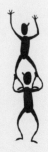

Abutment supported implant restorations are built with three components including an implant body, an abutment, and the restoration.

Implant supported restorations have only two components: the implant body and the restoration.

Implant-abutment supported restorations may be supported by an intermediary abutment, or directly by the implant body.

Examples

Screw Retained Abutment

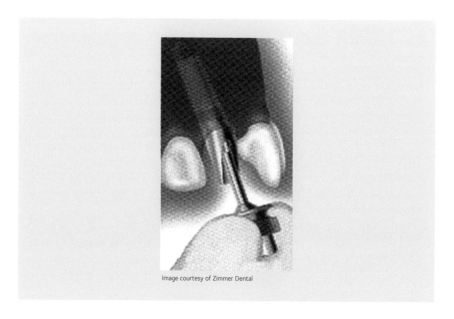

Image courtesy of Zimmer Dental

This illustration of a screw retained abutment shows how the abutment is a separate component that is attached to the implant body prior to placement of the final restorative prosthesis. There are a variety of abutments available (e.g., screw retained; "UCLA") there are only two procedure codes for implant abutments:

> **D6056** **prefabricated abutment – includes placement**
>
> **D6057** **custom abutment – includes placement**

Abutment Supported Porcelain/Ceramic Crown

Selection of the procedure code for the final restorative prostheses will be based on the type of materials used in fabrication and the nomenclature will begin with "abutment supported."

Abutment supported prosthetics are attached directly to the abutment, not the implant body. This illustration shows a porcelain/ceramic crown being seated on a prefabricated abutment. The crown may be cemented or screw retained. Procedure codes are:

D6056 **prefabricated abutment – includes placement**

D6058 **abutment supported porcelain/ceramic crown**
A single crown restoration that is retained, supported and stabilized by an abutment on an implant; may be screw retained or cemented.

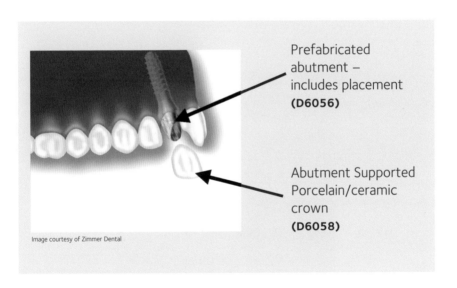

Prefabricated
abutment –
includes placement
(D6056)

Abutment Supported
Porcelain/ceramic
crown
(D6058)

Image courtesy of Zimmer Dental

Abutment Supported Fixed Partial Denture (FPD)

This illustration shows a fixed partial denture attached to two prefabricated abutments by screws. The abutments are attached to each implant body. Although available in a variety of shapes and sizes, prefabricated abutments would all be coded as D6056.

The applicable procedure codes in this example are:

D6069-71	**abutment supported retainer for porcelain fused to metal FPD (high noble, base or noble metal)**
D6240-42	**pontic – porcelain fused to metal (high noble, base or noble metal)**
D6056	**prefabricated abutment – includes placement**
D6010	**surgical placement of implant body: endosteal implant**

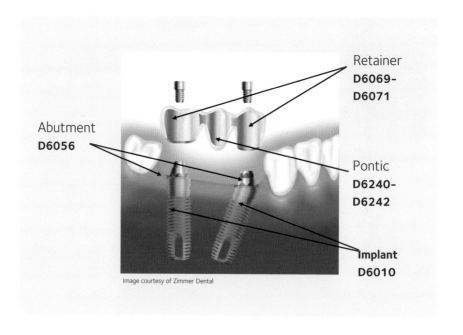

Image courtesy of Zimmer Dental

Implant Supported Crown

This is an illustration of a restoration attached directly to an implant body without use of an intermediary abutment. When a separate abutment is not utilized, the restorative prosthesis nomenclature will begin with "implant supported."

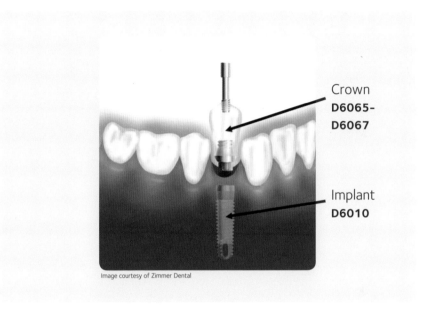

Crown
D6065–
D6067

Implant
D6010

Image courtesy of Zimmer Dental

Implant/Abutment Supported Prosthetics

The defining feature of this type of prosthesis is that there is not a direct correlation between implant positions and replacement teeth. Implant/abutment supported prosthetics always replace multiple teeth. They can replace a full complement of teeth (complete arch) or a partial arch, and may be removable, fixed or hybrid.

What's the difference?

It is not always easy to see the difference between an abutment supported fixed complete denture or an implant/abutment supported fixed complete denture.

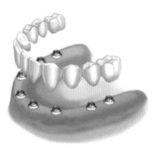

Prosthesis can either be screw-retained
or cement-retained.

The abutment supported fixed denture and the implant supported fixed denture both have a direct correlation between specific teeth and the implants that support them. The above prosthesis is fabricated as a fixed partial denture and would likewise be documented using fixed partial denture retainer codes from the *Code's* Implant Services category, and pontic codes from the Prosthodontics (fixed) category.

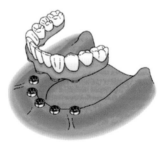

The implant/abutment supported fixed denture does not have a direct correlation between the implants and the teeth in the prosthesis. For this type of prosthesis, the replacement teeth are processed in denture acrylic and then seated and secured onto the abutments or implant bodies.

Implant/Abutment Supported Removable Denture

This is an illustration of a completely edentulous arch that is being restored with an abutment supported removable overdenture. Code D6053 would be used to document a removable complete overdenture whether supported directly by implants, or by intermediary abutments. In this example, prefabricated abutments will retain and stabilize the overdenture.

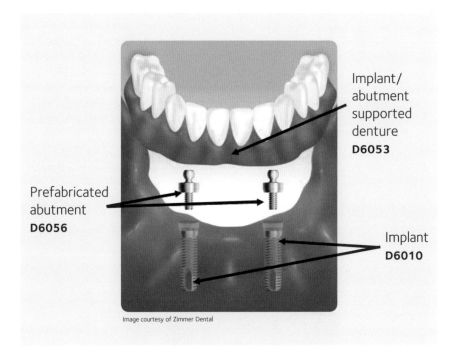

Implant/
abutment
supported
denture
D6053

Prefabricated
abutment
D6056

Implant
D6010

Image courtesy of Zimmer Dental

Prior to 2002, this prosthesis would have been documented as "D5860 overdenture – complete, by report" that is in the *Code's* removable prosthodontics category. D5860 continues to be used for tooth supported overdentures. With the version of the *Code* effective January 1, 2003, implant related overdentures are documented using the implant/abutment supported codes found in the Implant Services category.

Dental Implant Supported Connecting Bar

This illustration shows an abutment supported overdenture that utilizes a connecting bar. Connecting bars are retentive in nature, and can be utilized with rigid as well as resilient prosthetics. Hader® and Dolder® bar are two types of connecting bars. Connecting bars can be designed to use other types of retentive mechanisms, such as semi precision attachments.

Abutment supported connecting bars should be reported as:

> **D6055** **connecting bar – implant supported or abutment supported**
> Utilized to stabilize and anchor a prosthesis.

The entire connecting bar is reported as a single unit; however, an abutment would be documented for each implant that supports the connecting bar. Although the nomenclature says the connecting bar is "implant supported" the descriptor specifies that this procedure requires the use of abutments.

*"transmucosal" refers to the characteristic that these abutments connect the submucosal implant body to the supramucosal connecting bar. In fact, all abutments in the Code (**D6056 & D6057**) are transmucosal.*

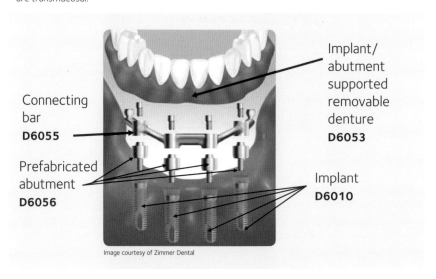

Connecting bar
D6055

Prefabricated abutment
D6056

Implant/abutment supported removable denture
D6053

Implant
D6010

Image courtesy of Zimmer Dental

It is also possible to construct a connecting bar that attaches directly to the implant bodies, but there are no specific procedure codes for such a device. In such cases it is necessary to document the bar using the code for unspecified implant procedures, **D6199,** which requires the inclusion of a narrative description.

Implant/Abutment Supported Fixed Denture

The following illustration combines elements of a complete overdenture with a fixed component and is sometimes referred to as a hybrid prostheses. This example would be documented as:

D6078 **implant/abutment supported fixed denture for completely edentulous arch**
A prosthesis that is retained, supported and stabilized by implants or abutments placed on implants, but does not have specific relationships between implant positions and replacement teeth; may be screw-retained or cemented; commonly referred to as a "hybrid prosthesis."

D6056 **prefabricated abutment – includes placement**
A connection to an implant that is a manufactured component usually made of machined high noble metal, titanium, titanium alloy or ceramic. Modification of a prefabricated abutment may be necessary, and is accomplished by altering its shape using dental burs/diamonds.

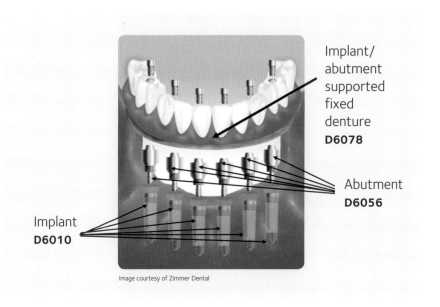

Implant/ abutment supported fixed denture **D6078**

Abutment **D6056**

Implant **D6010**

Image courtesy of Zimmer Dental

Summary – Choosing the Right Codes

Abutment supported implant prosthetics are documented with at least three procedure codes.

1. Implant body

2. Abutment

3. Prosthesis Single Crown / FPD / RPD)

When the prosthesis is a fixed partial denture (FPD) the pontic codes are located in the Prosthetics (fixed) Category of Service (**D6205-D6252**). A connector bar, when used, would be documented as D6055.

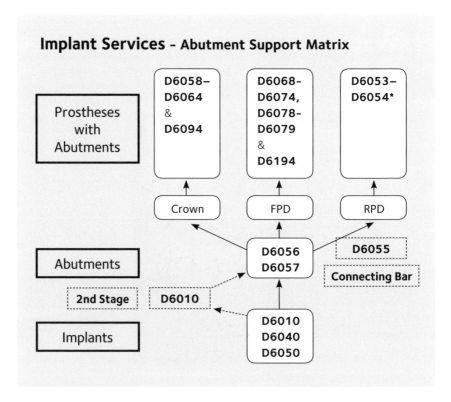

Implant Services - Abutment Support Matrix

* Codes **D6053, D6054, D6078 & D6079** have "implant/abutment" in their nomenclatures, which means that they are also found in the following implant support matrix.

Implant supported prosthetics are documented with at least two procedure codes.

1. Implant body

2. Prosthesis (Single Crown / FPD / RPD)

When the prosthesis is a fixed partial denture (FPD) or removable partial denture (RPD) with pontics, the pontic codes are located in the Prosthetics (fixed) Category of Service (**D6205-D6252**). A connector bar, when used, would be documented as D6199.

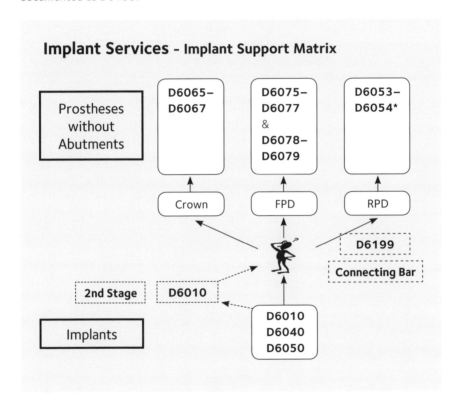

Implant Services - Implant Support Matrix

* Codes **D6053, D6054, D6078** & **D6079** have "implant/abutment" in their nomenclatures, which means that they are also found in the preceding abutment support matrix.

Coding Exercises – Day-to-Day Code Use

5

CDT
Companion

Chapter 5
Coding Exercises –
Day-to-Day Code Use

This chapter contains a number of exercises designed to help you practice your coding skills and are based on "real life" situations. These exercises have been devised to illustrate varied aspects of the *Code*. The answers are intended to demonstrate possible coding solutions for the situations described. Scenarios and their solutions have been developed to reflect common and accepted practices, but may not reflect the way your office would manage a given situation. The dentist who treats a patient is the person who can best determine appropriate treatment and what codes will best describe it.

These exercises and their solutions are not to be considered legal advice or a guarantee that individual payer contracts will follow this assistance.

Use these exercises to get a better understanding of the principles of reporting using the *Code*. Since the exercises cover subjects from many different aspects of the *Code* it is likely that some exercises will be more applicable to your particular situation than others. All the exercises, including those that involve procedures you may not usually report, may be of value since the principles that are demonstrated can often be applied to other areas of the *Code*.

Using the analogy of the *Code* as a language, this section could be considered "conversational" training. It allows you to apply coded "vocabulary" and "grammar" to commonly encountered situations. Space has been provided for you to record your own answers to each question. Compare your solutions to those provided. The most benefit and satisfaction will come from engaging in the "conversation" yourself, rather than just "listening."

Remember,

- "Code for what you do" is the fundamental rule to apply in all coding situations.

- The *Code* is a language that allows efficient communication between parties, but like any language, the precision and nuances of what is communicated can be lost in translation.

- When using the *Code* to accomplish your reporting goals, there are times when similar things can be translated in different ways, therefore the most precise communication takes place when you have a complete understanding of the available vocabulary.

- The existence of a procedure code does not mean that the procedure is a covered or reimbursed benefit in a dental benefit plan.

The exercises vary in their complexity; however, whether an individual finds a particular exercise difficult will depend upon scope of their experience using the *Code*.

Keep in mind that the terminology the dental team and others use to describe various procedures may depend on when and where they practice or went to school. In many cases, these terms are used interchangeably, for example:

- Maryland Bridge = Bonded Bridge

- Bridge or Bridgework = Fixed Partial Denture (FPD)

- Abutment = Fixed or Removable Partial Denture Retainer

- Abutment = Implant-supported intermediary component of some implant restorative systems

- Retainer =Teeth that serve as support for a fixed partial denture

- Retainer = orthodontic treatment maintenance appliance

- "Flipper" = Interim Partial Denture

If you have difficulty finding a code, consider whether there may be another way to describe the procedure. The CDT manual's glossary and alphabetic index are likely to be helpful in these situations.

Dental procedure codes vs. medical procedure codes

The *Code* is the source for procedure codes used when submitting claims to dental benefit plans on either the ADA Dental Claim Form or the HIPAA standard electronic dental claim transaction. There may be times when a dentist's services are submitted to a patient's medical benefit plan. When this happens not only is there a different claim form, there are also different procedure codes that must be used.

Medical procedure codes come from two sources, the American Medical Association's Current Procedure Terminology (CPT) code set and the federal government's Healthcare Common Procedure Code Set (HCPCS). When selecting a medical procedure code the rule of thumb is to first look at the CPT code set to determine if there is an appropriate code to use. If there is none, a HCPCS code may be used.

Two of the following coding exercises, #8 and #15, illustrate how CPT or HCPCS procedure codes may be used. There is much more information about these two code sets in the discussion of medical claim submission and dental to medical procedure cross coding that is in Chapter 10.

Coding Exercise #1

Topical fluoride treatments – preventive; sensitivity; caries risk

Three friends decided to visit their dentist together. They all had their teeth cleaned and checked and each one had fluoride varnish applied to their teeth at the end of the visit, but when they compared their statements afterward, the dentist had used a different code for each one. Can you match the code with the appropriate application?

1) Bob had never had a cavity, which he attributed to the great preventive care he had always received. This included regular cleanings and topical fluoride treatments.

2) Bill had not had a cavity in many years, but since his last visit there were a number of teeth that had become sensitive. The doctor had applied varnish to each of those teeth to make them less sensitive.

3) Ben had gone for years without a cavity, but this visit he had decay on the roots of two teeth and there were others that looked suspicious. He had recently started taking an anti-depressant medication that left his mouth dry, and found that sucking on candy made him feel more comfortable. The dentist suggested that he might need to have the varnish applied again in a few weeks.

Solutions:

Bob:

> **D1204   topical application of fluoride – adult**

Bob just got his usual preventive application of fluoride. The *Code* does not specify the type or delivery method of the fluoride application, so this code is appropriate for gels, foams, aqueous solutions, and in this case fluoride varnish.

Bill:

> **D9910   application of desensitizing medicament**

The original FDA-approved usage for fluoride varnish was treatment of sensitivity. **D9910** is used to code for a number of different formulations and techniques that treat tooth sensitivity, including fluoride varnish. Bill had multiple teeth treated, but this code is typically used on a "per visit" basis when fluoride is the desensitizing agent.

Ben:

> **D1206   topical fluoride varnish; therapeutic application for moderate
> to high risk caries patients**

This new code is specifically for fluoride varnish and recognizes that patients with a moderate to high risk of developing cavities due to caries may require a different treatment regimen. Ben was determined to be at higher risk due to his recent caries history, including root caries, medication he was taking and higher risk behaviors like sucking on candy.

Coding Exercise #2

Patient age 11 – evaluation and preventive services

A new patient, age 11, was seen for a first exam, cleaning, and fluoride application. During the exam the dentist noted that the erupting tooth #4 was impinging on the band loop spacer cemented to #3 and decided to remove it.

1) How might this visit be coded?

2) What if the same patient was not new and the doctor had placed the space maintainer two years ago. How would this encounter be coded?

3) What would change if the patient was 12 years old?

4) What if the patient only had permanent teeth?

Solutions:

1) The new patient visit could be coded as:

D0150	comprehensive oral evaluation – new or established patient
D1120	prophylaxis – child
D1203	topical application of fluoride – child
D1555	removal of fixed space maintainer

In this scenario, codes **D1120** and **D1203** were used because the codes that combined prophylaxis and fluoride application (**D1201** and **D1205**) deleted from the *Code* as of January 1, 2007. **D1555 removal of fixed space maintainer** is a code that was added effective the same date.

2) If the patient was a previous patient of record, the visit might be coded as:

D0120	periodic oral evaluation
D1120	prophylaxis – child
D1203	topical application of fluoride – child

The exam, in this case, would be periodic (**D0120**) because the patient was seen previously, but the other codes remain the same. It should be noted that it would not be appropriate to use code **D1555** because its descriptor specifies that this procedure code is for use by a dentist who did not place the space maintainer.

3) Both the adult codes and the child codes can be used for patients with transitional dentitions regardless of age. Patient age is not a part of the codes' nomenclatures or descriptors. ADA policy recommends that dental benefit determinations should be based on dental development rather than patient age.

ADA Policy: Age of "Child" (1991:635)

The ADA Policy adopted by the House of Delegates states that:
   • Benefits should be based on stage of dentition
   • If a plan cannot recognize stage of dentition, age 12 should be recognized as the age of an adult, in terms of dentition (with the exclusion of treatment for orthodontics and sealants).

The prophylaxis codes are dentition-specific rather than age-specific. Some third-party payers have restrictions in their contracts that limit available benefits based on age, not stage of dentition. Most dental benefit plans specify an age between 12 and 21 when the patient is considered an adult.

4) Regardless of age, patients with a permanent dentition are most appropriately coded using the adult codes (**D1110** & **D1204**). In this case, if third party payers substitute a procedure for a child during processing, it would be considered downcoding.

From the CDT manual glossary:

downcoding: A practice of third-party payers in which the benefit code has been changed to a less complex and/or lower cost procedure than was reported, except where delineated in contract agreements.

Coding Exercise #3

Child under three – evaluation and parent counseling, and preventive services

Dr. Thomas had been preparing himself for something new, but much of what he did at 10-month-old Katie's appointment, he had been doing routinely. He knew that the American Academy of Pediatric Dentistry and the ADA advise that children should have their first dental visit within six months of the eruption of the first primary tooth. However, he had a hard time thinking of children Katie's age, as patients.

In the past, Dr. Thomas had given new parents education regarding diet, proper use of bottles, and cleaning those new "baby" teeth, but had never really counted that as "billable" time. Recently however, Dr. Thomas attended a workshop where he learned about the significance of early prevention and a procedure code to report these early childhood encounters.

Dr. Thomas performed an intraoral examination while mom restrained Katie's forehead in her lap. The dentist was able to determine that Katie had maxillary and mandibular primary central incisors and that they were free of decay. He also removed plaque using an ultra-soft toothbrush and applied fluoride varnish. Dr. Thomas explained to Katie's mother how to use a wash cloth or soft brush to remove plaque each day and the importance of getting Katie to go to sleep without a bottle. They discussed foods that can lead to decay and recommended that she return in a year for an exam after most of the primary teeth have erupted.

To summarize, this is what occurred during the office visit:
- Oral examination
- Toothbrush deplaquing
- Fluoride varnish
- Discussion of diet and preventive care with her mother

1) How would you code this visit?

2) How could you code on Katie's next visit?

3) Is there more than one possibility for coding the fluoride varnish?

Solutions:

1) Katie's initial visit to Dr. Thomas could be coded using:

D0145   **oral evaluation for a patient under three years of age and counseling with primary caregiver**

D1120   **prophylaxis – child**

D1203   **topical application of fluoride – child**

> The "tiny tots" evaluation code (**D0145**):
> - has both diagnostic and preventive characteristics
> - is specifically for children under 3 years of age
> - includes an evaluation of oral conditions, history, & caries susceptibility
> - includes development of an oral hygiene regimen
> - always includes counseling the primary caregiver or parent

2) Either the "tiny tots" evaluation code (**D0145**) or the periodic evaluation (**D0120**) could be used for Katie's next visit. There is nothing in **D0145** that precludes its use for another visit, as long as the patient is still under three years of age and all the components of the procedure are completed. The periodic exam might be appropriate as the primary dentition develops and if the other criteria are not met. The prophylaxis and fluoride would remain the same.

3) A child's fluoride varnish application may be coded using the traditional child application code (**D1203**) or, if caries risk is determined to be moderate to high, the new fluoride varnish code (**D1206**). Since Dr. Thomas was not planning to see Katie for one year, this exercise assumed that she was not at moderate to high risk for caries. See exercise #1 for more details on the different codes applicable to fluoride varnish.

Coding Exercise #4

Radiographs – What constitutes a full mouth series (periapicals, bitewings and panoramic films)?

Here are three radiographic scenarios: How would you code them?

Betty is missing all second and third molars. The office takes ten periapical x-rays: three upper anterior, three lower anterior and one posterior in each quadrant.

Barbara has all her teeth and has impacted partially erupted third molars. The office takes a panoramic x-ray and four posterior bitewings.

Becky has a maxillary full denture and fourteen mandibular teeth. The office takes four periapicals of the upper edentulous ridge, seven periapicals of the lower arch and four posterior bitewings.

Solutions:

A change to the *Code on Dental Procedures and Nomenclature* effective January 1, 2009 added a descriptor to procedure code **D0210** that defined a complete mouth series of radiographic images. The descriptor is based on the glossary definition found in the FDA publication, *The Selection of Patients for X-Ray Examinations: Dental Radiographic Examinations:*

> "A set of intraoral radiographs usually consisting of 14 to 22 periapical and posterior bitewing films intended to display the crowns and roots of all teeth, periapical areas, and alveolar bone crest."

With that in mind, the scenarios in the exercise might be coded as follows:

Betty:
If the radiographs display the crowns and roots of all teeth, periapical areas and alveolar bone crest, the full mouth series procedure code would be appropriate. According to the Code Revision Committee code D0210 includes bitewings when indicated, but bitewings are not a required component of this procedure.

D0210	**intraoral – complete series (including bitewings)**
	A radiographic survey of the whole mouth, usually consisting of 14-22 periapical and posterior bitewing images intended to display the crowns and roots of all teeth, periapical areas and alveolar bone.

If the radiographs do not display all these structures, the applicable procedure codes are:

D0220   **intraoral – periapical first film** (reported once)

D0230   **intraoral – periapical each additional film** (reported nine times)

Barbara:

D0330   **panoramic film**

D0274   **bitewings – four films**

Since a panoramic film is not intraoral, this combination could not correctly be reported as a full mouth series, although the ADA Council on Dental Benefit Programs receives many calls that it is often downcoded this way by third-party payers.

From the CDT manual glossary:

downcoding: A practice of third-party payers in which the benefit code has been changed to a less complex and/or lower cost procedure than was reported, except where delineated in contract agreements.

Becky:

D0210   **intraoral – complete series (including bitewings)**
A radiographic survey of the whole mouth, usually consisting of 14-22 periapical and posterior bitewing images intended to display the crowns and roots of all teeth, periapical areas and alveolar bone.

This situation, while not the most common scenario, does meet all the criteria of both the *Code* and the FDA guidelines and is correctly coded as a full mouth series.

Regardless of the benefit plan possessed by a patient, the reporting of performed procedures should always reflect what treatment was actually provided. Alternate payment provisions may apply, but the third-party payers should send statements to patients and providers alike that explain why an alternate benefit was provided.

Dentists who have signed provider agreements with third-party payers should check their contracts to see if there are provisions that apply to this situation.

Quick Quiz #1: "partial" prophylaxis

Q: Many adult patients have less than a full complement of teeth. How do you code for "partial" prophylaxis, for example, when a patient has one edentulous arch and another partially edentulous arch?

A: In these cases, **D1110 prophylaxis–adult** should be used.

Neither the nomenclature nor descriptor for this code contain any language that precludes its use for less than a full mouth procedure.

Quick Quiz #2: Post and cores for single crowns and for fixed partial dentures

Q: There are post and core codes found in both the restorative category and the fixed prosthodontics category. Which is the correct code to use?

A: The code reported is based on the treatment plan.

When the final restoration will be a single unit:

D2952	**post and core in addition to crown, indirectly fabricated**
D2954	**prefabricated post and core in addition to crown**

When the final restoration will be a multiple unit fixed bridge:

D6970	**post and core in addition to fixed partial denture retainer, indirectly fabricated**
D6972	**prefabricated post and core in addition to fixed partial denture retainer**

Coding Exercise #5

Fractured tooth – after hours visit and the final restoration

"I broke my front tooth Doc" was not what Dr. Anderson wanted to hear on Saturday, a day the office was usually closed, but she agreed to meet the patient. On examination, tooth #8 appeared to have a fractured mesial-incisal angle and lost a mesial composite restoration, but it "didn't hurt." Dr. Anderson appreciated that the tooth was not too attractive in its current state and it was irritating the patient's tongue. She removed enough tooth structure to fit a polycarbonate temporary crown, which she cemented. Dr. Anderson told the patient that the tooth would need a porcelain-fused-to-metal crown (PFM), but this could be done at a scheduled appointment during regular office hours.

1) How could you code for this after hours visit?

When the patient returned to the office, Dr. Anderson removed the temporary crown. Following caries excavation, she determined that the tooth required some replacement of lost structure to achieve proper strength and retention for the crown. She used one threaded titanium pin and a bonded resin core material to restore the tooth, and then prepared and took an impression for a PFM. The PFM was fabricated using an alloy containing gold 15%, Palladium 25 % and Platinum 10%.

2) How would this visit during regular office hours be coded?

Solutions:

1) Dr. Anderson's Saturday services could be coded as:

D0140   **limited oral evaluation – problem focused**

D2970   **temporary crown (fractured tooth)**

D9440   **office visit – after regularly scheduled hours**

The code for a temporary crown (**D2970**) was deleted from the *Code* as of January 1, 2005, but was returned effective January 1, 2007 along with a change to the descriptor. It is appropriately used for this emergency situation, but should not be used for temporization during laboratory fabrication of a new crown.

The after-hours office visit code (**D9440**) is from the adjunctive services section of the *Code* and can be reported in addition to the other services performed at that appointment. This service may not be a covered benefit under some dental benefits plans.

2) The next visit during regular office hours might be coded as:

D2950   **core buildup, including any pins**

D2752   **crown – porcelain fused to noble metal**

Replacement of tooth structure that is more than simply filling undercuts is appropriately reported using the code for a core buildup (**D2950**). The retentive pin that was placed is included in this code. If a material is used only to eliminate undercuts, usually termed a base, it is included in the crown preparation procedure.

The code for a PFM utilizing a noble metal (**D2752**) rather than a high noble metal (**D2750**) was selected because the alloy used in the crown contains more than 25% but less than 60% noble metals.

Coding Exercise #6

Indirect restorations – laboratory crowns vs. in-office CAD/CAM crowns

Dr. Miller loved his new CAD/CAM machine and was using it for more procedures all the time. Right now the machine was hard at work in the other room, milling an esthetic post and core for tooth #8. When it was competed, he would cement the post and prepare the tooth for the final all-ceramic crown, which would be milled with the same machine minutes later. Dr. Miller's patients appreciated the esthetics of this all-ceramic restorative solution and the convenience of having these fabricated while they waited. What Dr. Miller appreciated most, at least when it was time to write the monthly check for the lease, was that his capable staff would know exactly how to code for these procedures.

1) How would you do it?

Across the hall, Dr. Goldsmith didn't even have a computer in his office, but he appreciated his lab technician's fine casting skills as he, coincidentally, was also restoring #8 with a post and core. He cemented the fine cast gold post and core that he had taken an impression for at the patient's last visit. Now he took the final impression for a porcelain jacket crown which would be fabricated using a traditional porcelain layering technique by the ceramist at his favorite lab. What he appreciated most, at least when it was time to write the monthly check to the lab, was that his capable staff would know exactly how to code for these procedures.

2) How would you do it?

Solutions:

1&2) Both Dr. Miller's and Dr. Goldsmith's treatments would be coded as:

D2952   **post and core indirectly fabricated – in addition to crown**

D2740   **crown – porcelain/ceramic substrate**

Code **D2952** was changed effective January 1, 2007, to include indirectly fabricated posts and cores including those milled using CAD/CAM fabricators. Although Dr. Miller did not take an impression, the milled post and core was custom fabricated using an indirect method. Since casting metal posts and cores is also an indirect method, **D2952** continues to be the correct code for Dr. Goldsmith's treatment.

An all ceramic crown, whether milled or built up and vacuum-fired, is coded using **D2740**.

Coding Exercise #7

Multiple restorations on the same tooth

Dr. King had warned Louie that poor hygiene plus braces spelled trouble, and sure enough, the bitewings he received from the orthodontist told the tale. Just below the contact between nearly every posterior tooth, a pair of dark triangles indicated incipient decay. Dr. King hoped they would not all need to be restored, so he recommended a monthly application of fluoride varnish until Louie's next cleaning appointment. Unfortunately, there were several that would need immediate restoration. Tooth #14 received separate MO and DO restorations and #19 had an MOD and a buccal pit restoration. All the restorations were done with composite resin.

How would you code for the procedures on this visit?

The next month, Dr. King focused on Louie's right where the buccal surface of #28, below where the bracket had been bonded, had an area of decayed enamel that required restoration. He removed the caries and demineralized enamel, but discovered that he had not penetrated into the dentin. The cavity was restored with composite resin.

How would you code for this procedure?

Solutions:

Appointment 1:

Since it is clear that Louie is at high risk for caries, the code for the therapeutic application of fluoride varnish would be the appropriate code for this preventive intervention:

> **D1206** **topical fluoride varnish; therapeutic application for moderate to high caries risk patients**

Restorations #14:

> **D2392** **resin-based composite – two surface, posterior**

Reported twice (MO and DO)

Restorations #19:

> **D2393** **resin-based composite – three surface, posterior**
>
> **D2391** **resin-based composite – one surface, posterior**

Dental plans may have clauses that restrict coverage on the same surface twice on the same date of service, and an alternate benefit provision may be applied. For example, payers often downcode separate restorations by recoding them as a single multiple surface restoration. Nevertheless, when individual restorations on the same teeth are done, there is nothing in the *Code* to indicate that it is not appropriate to report them separately.

Appointment 2:

There is not a specific code to report a one surface posterior resin restoration on smooth surfaces when the tooth preparation does not extend into dentin. When there is not a specific procedure code that is applicable to the service, then the Dnn99 codes (unspecified procedure, by report) can be used. In this case, **"D2999 unspecified restorative procedure, by report"** may be reported. All "by report" procedure codes are expected to include a supporting narrative that explains the service provided.

Some third-party payers will consider this procedure to be a sealant (**D1351**).

Coding Exercise #8

Sleep apnea appliance

A dentist's husband was keeping her up all night with his snoring so she made him a sleep apnea appliance with maxillary and mandibular components that dock to prevent closure of the airway. She struggled with recording the procedure because there did not appear to be a code for a snoring appliance, and she was even uncertain about what category of service this would fall under, if she was going to use a "by report" code.

Is there a way to code for this procedure?

Solutions:

Many people are unaware that the Maxillofacial Prosthetics category includes a number of non-orthodontic adjunctive treatment appliances.

There is not a specific code for the sleep apnea device, but because of its similarity to these other appliances in the Maxillofacial Prosthetics category, it would probably be appropriate to use code

D5999 **unspecified maxillofacial prosthesis, by report.**

If you were seeking benefits for this type of appliance, The American Academy of Dental Sleep Medicine (AADSM) suggests that they are most appropriately billed to a medical plan.

The following HCPCS Level II code is a possibility:

E0486 **Oral device/appliance used to reduce upper airway collapsibility, adjustable or non-adjustable, custom fabricated, includes fitting and adjustment.**

More information on filing claims to medical plans can be found in the Dental/Medical Cross Coding section (Chapter 10) of this manual.

Coding Exercise #9

Dates of service for prosthodontic treatment and for endodontic treatment

Mitch and Dr. Kronos had a regular date for an entire month. Mitch traveled for work all week, but returned for the weekend and spent the day every Monday catching up at home. When Mitch needed some more extensive dental treatment he scheduled to have an appointment every Monday for a month. Thanks to Dr. Kronos' extremely efficient lab, they were able to finish all of Mitch's treatment that month.

November 2010

Sun	Mon	Tue	Wed	Thu	Fri	Sat
	1 Dr. Kronos	2	3	4	5	6
7	8 Dr. Kronos	9	10	11	12	13
14	15 Dr. Kronos	16	17	18	19	20
21	22 Dr. Kronos	23	24	25	26	27
28	29 Dr. Kronos	30				

ADA®

This is what they did each visit:

1st: Began root canal treatment #20

8th: Completed root canal treatment #20,
        Prepared and took an impression for a cast gold post/core

15th: Cemented cast post/core,
        Prepared and took an impression for a PFM surveyed crown #20

22nd: Cemented crown #20
        Prepared and took an impression for an immediate transitional lower
        removable partial denture (replacing #18, 19, 29, 30, 31)

29th: Extracted teeth #18, 32
        Delivered immediate transitional lower removable partial denture

Which date should be reported for each procedure?

Solutions:

ADA policy encourages third party payers to count the date of impression as the date of service in fixed and removable prosthetic cases.[1] However, some state laws and third party processing policies and contract provisions, specify the completion date as the date of service. The ADA also recommends the date of completion as the date of service for endodontic treatment.[2]

Ethics dictate consistency in the way we treat patients with or without dental benefits. Regional preferences and customs may also play a role. Finally, particular procedures may naturally create exceptions to the rules based on laboratory commitments or correlated procedures, like extractions prior to delivery. You should weigh all these factors when determining the date of service, emphasizing consistency and compliance with applicable rules.

The following are recommended reporting dates are based on current ADA policies:

Root Canal – 8th: Although the largest portion of the procedure may be done on the first appointment, the recommended reporting date is following completion.

Post/Core – 8th: There is not a specific policy relating to reporting of indirect post and cores, but the impression date would be consistent with other indirect procedures.

PFM crown – 15th: While ADA policy recommends the impression date, a number of states have laws that dictate that the completion date is the date of service for dental prosthetics. Carriers may also request the cementation date for processing claims.

Partial denture – 22nd: Although some teeth that will be replaced with the immediate partial denture have not yet been extracted, generally the impression date would still be considered the date of service.

Extractions – 29th: Extractions are always reported on the date they are performed. It is never appropriate to report extractions earlier on immediate denture cases.

[1] **ADA Policy Payment of Prosthodontic Treatment (1989:547)**
Resolved, that the Council on Dental Benefit Programs encourages all third-party payers to recognize the preparation date as the date of service, that is, payment date, for fixed prosthodontic treatment, and be it further
Resolved, that the Council on Dental Benefit Programs encourages all third-party payers to recognize the final impression date as the date of service, that is payment date, for removable prosthodontic treatment.

[2] **ADA Policy Eligibility and Payment Dates for Endodontic Treatment (1994:674)**
Resolved, that the American Dental Association through its Council on Dental Benefit Programs, encourages all third-party payers to recognize the date that endodontic therapy is begun as the eligibility date for coverage for endodontic therapy, and be it further
Resolved, that the Association, through its Council on Dental Benefit Programs, encourages all third-party payers to recognize the completion date as the date of service, that is, the payment date, for endodontic therapy.

Quick Quiz #3a: Radiographs and Endodontic treatment

Q: Can we code for the radiographs and other diagnostic procedures we do prior to endodontic treatment?

A: The descriptor of endodontic therapy states that coding for endodontic procedures **D3310, D3320,** and **D3330** does not include diagnostic evaluation and necessary diagnostic radiographs/images. It is appropriate to report an evaluation or diagnostic radiographs/images when clinical circumstances dictate these procedures are necessary. There is also a code for pulp vitality tests, **D0460**.

Quick Quiz #3b: Stimulating formation of a root apex

Q: What is the code for an endodontic procedure to stimulate the formation of a root apex in an incompletely developed tooth that does require complete root canal therapy?

A: Apexogenesis is vital pulp therapy performed to encourage continued physiological formation and development of the tooth root. To report this procedure, use the procedure code that was added effective January 1, 2009 - **D3222 partial pulpotomy for apexogenesis - permanent tooth with incomplete root development.**

Quick Quiz #4a: New patient for Orthodontic services

Q: An orthodontic office has a patient in for an examination, radiographs, photographs and impressions for study models, and then has them return for a second appointment where the doctor presents the details of the treatment plan and answers questions. Is there a way to code for each of these visits?

A: The initial visit might be coded with:

    D0150 **comprehensive oral evaluation**
    D0340 **cephalometric film**
    D0350 **oral/facial photographic images**
    D0470 **diagnostic casts**

This, of course, would be dependent on the kind of evaluation and radiographs that were actually done.

For the second visit you might use code **D9450 case presentation, detailed and extensive treatment planning** since the procedure: was not performed on the same day as an evaluation; was performed for an established patient; involved the consideration of a number of diagnostic aids; and will require treatment over an extended period of time.

Quick Quiz #4b: Clear aligners

Q: Clear dental aligners such as ClearCorrect™, Invisalign® or Red White & Blue® seem so different from conventional orthodontic therapy. Is there a different way to code this kind of treatment?

A: There is no unique procedure code for such devices. Orthodontic procedures are reported based on the practitioner's diagnosis and treatment plan for the patient. Depending on the treatment objective and stage of dentition, codes are available for primary, transitional, adolescent and adult dentitions that are treatment planned for limited, interceptive or comprehensive orthodontic treatment.

Coding Exercise #10

Oral cancer – an enhanced examination

An oral cancer evaluation is included in the descriptors of both of the comprehensive oral evaluations (**D0150** and **D0180**) and the periodic oral evaluation (**D0120**). Visual inspection using operatory lighting and palpation are the techniques that are frequently used in routine oral cancer evaluations. A dentist may decide that patients with increased cancer risk factors should also receive an enhanced oral cancer examination, one that is more extensive than a routine oral cancer screening and may include the use of additional diagnostic aids.

How could this dentist report this added procedure?

Solutions:

There is not an independent code for an enhanced oral cancer examination, but there is a code that can be used when some type of staining or similar procedure is performed:

D0431   **adjunctive pre-diagnostic test that aids in detection of mucosal abnormalities including premalignant and malignant lesions, not to include cytology or biopsy procedures**

This code would be used to report the use of chemiluminescent testing (e.g. Vizilite®) or any intra-oral staining technique (e.g. toluidine blue).

If the additional procedures are not described by **D0431** the dentist could use:

D0999   **unspecified diagnostic procedure, by report**

D0999 can be used to report any diagnostic procedure which does not seem to be included in the *Code*. Use of this code requires the inclusion of a narrative that describes the service that was provided.

Coding Exercise #11

Orthognathic surgery planning

An oral & maxillofacial surgery office recently installed a cone beam radiography machine (Cone Beam CT). It was used to treatment plan some anticipated orthognathic surgery for a patient. Following image capture, several axial and lateral views were consulted to plan the surgery. A panoramic view was also produced to send to the patient's orthodontist.

After consultation with the orthodontist, the surgeon constructed a 3D virtual model, which they viewed together on the computer, to properly locate a temporary implant to anchor the orthodontic appliance. The virtual model could be manipulated on the screen to allow them to visualize other anatomical structures in the area and their relationship to the teeth to determine the ideal location to place the implant.

A transmucosal endosseous implant was placed as a temporary fixation device for the patient's braces. The temporary implant will be removed when orthodontic treatment is completed.

How could you code:

- The initial treatment planning visit?
  (includes initial scan, coronal & sagittal views, and panoramic view)

- Subsequent consultation?
  (3D virtual model)

- Temporary implant placement requiring surgical flap?

Solutions:

Treatment plan visit:

> **D0360**   **cone beam ct – craniofacial data capture**
>
> **D0362**   **cone beam – two-dimensional image reconstruction using existing data, includes multiple images**

These codes were added effective January 1, 2007 specifically to report procedures related to the new cone beam imaging technology. The initial image capture also includes two-dimensional sectional (tomographic) views from the axial (coronal or frontal) and lateral (sagittal) planes. The cone beam technology also allows oblique sectional views in these planes.

The panoramic view is actually a reconstruction that is a two-dimensional composite image made from various sectional planes, so the two-dimensional reconstruction code is used.

Consultation visit:

> **D0363**   **cone beam – three-dimensional image reconstruction using existing data, includes multiple images**

The virtual model is really a three-dimensional image which is again reconstructed from data in all the sectional planes. In this case the code for the three-dimensional reconstruction would be used.

Temporary implant placement:

> **D7293**   **surgical placement: temporary surgical anchorage device requiring surgical flap**

Temporary implants also represent a new kind of technology for which codes were added effective January 1, 2007. The correct code to use for this type of implant depends upon whether it will be used for fixation or an interim restoration. In this case, the implant is being used as a fixation device for orthodontics, so the correct code comes from the *Code's* Oral & Maxillofacial Surgery category. (Note: if the temporary implant does not require a surgical flap, the correct code would be **D7294**.)

Cone Beam CT technology

The Cone Beam CT machine looks very much like a panoramic x-ray machine, but utilizes a cone-shaped beam and a curved sensor to capture a volumetric "image" resulting in "voxels" rather than pixels.

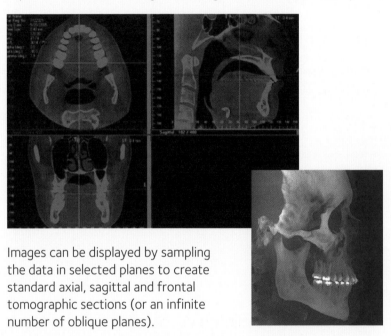

Images can be displayed by sampling the data in selected planes to create standard axial, sagittal and frontal tomographic sections (or an infinite number of oblique planes).

The data can also be used to reconstruct two dimensional images resembling familiar panoramic, cephalometric or periapical radiographs, and three dimensional views or milled models that can be manipulated.

There are numerous dental applications including surgical preparation and diagnosis, implants and orthodontics.

Rapid acceptance of this new technology necessitated the adoption of codes for the Cone Beam CT. Because of the unique data capture and manipulations possible, three codes were added to provide the dental community with a method for reporting these procedures.

Images courtesy Imaging Sciences International, Inc. www.i-cat.com

Quick Quiz #5a: Removing a temporary implant

Q: How do you code for the removal of a temporary implant?

A: The descriptors for all temporary implant codes (**D6012, D7292, D7293** and **D7294**) specify that removal is included with the initial placement.

Quick Quiz #5b: Cone Beam cephalometric view

Q: How do you code for a Cephalometric view reconstructed from a Cone Beam CT scan?

A: While the Cephalometric view resembles a lateral (sagittal) sectional view, it is in fact a composite of a number of sagittal sections and would therefore be considered a two-dimensional reconstruction. Use code **D0362**.

Coding Exercise #12

Modifying an existing partial denture after an extraction

Rufus came to see Dr. Lancaster complaining that he could not wear his upper partial because of some loose, painful teeth. Dr. Lancaster determined that he had a well-designed maxillary removable partial denture and that it was not in bad shape. The partial replaced teeth #2, 3, 4, and 14, with clasps on teeth #5, 13 and 15. His evaluation indicated that tooth #13 had Class III mobility due to advanced periodontal bone loss; #12 was fractured and decayed so that only a small piece of root remained exposed. Tooth #15 had a fractured MOBL silver amalgam restoration with a fair amount of recurrent decay. Dr. Lancaster suggested the following treatment plan:

- Extraction of teeth #12 and #13
- Addition of teeth #12 and #13 to the partial
- Add an additional clasp to the partial for retention on tooth #11.
- Construct a full cast noble metal crown tooth #15 which will be made to fit the existing clasp

How would each of these procedures be coded?

Solutions:

Extractions:

D7140   extraction, erupted tooth or exposed root (elevation and/or forceps removal)

Both the routine extraction of #13 and the root tip removal of #12 could be coded using **D7140**. If the root tip removal required the laying of a mucoperiosteal flap and bone removal, the appropriate code for surgical extractions is **D7210.**

Addition of teeth to partial:

D5650   add tooth to existing partial denture

This code would be used once for each tooth added and generally requires reporting of the tooth number.

Addition of clasp to partial:

D5660   add clasp to existing partial denture

There is a single code for the addition of a clasp to a partial, whether it is wrought wire and processed or cast and soldered.

Crown to fit partial:

D2790   crown – full cast high noble metal

D2971   additional procedures to construct new crown under existing partial denture framework

When a crown is constructed to fit an existing partial denture the code for a regular crown is selected based on the material from which it is fabricated. The additional procedures required to allow the crown to accommodate the existing clasp are coded using **D2971.**

Coding Exercise #13

Implant supported denture for an edentulous patient

Joe had been wearing dentures for over 40 years. He had done very well for most of those years with only the occasional reline, but the last couple had been pretty miserable. He had been using an adhesive to glue them in since the first day after his last reline and even that wasn't working very well. Dr. Benton had been recommending implants for nearly five years, but Joe had resisted because he felt he was too old for the expense. Now he had come to the conclusion that he really needed to do something. Dr. Benton recommended the following:

- Four endosseous implants
- An abutment supported connecting bar with Hader® and ERA® attachments
- A new mandibular complete denture (overdenture)

How would you code for these procedures?

Solutions:

The prosthetic treatment described in this exercise is an implant/abutment supported denture which has three components:

Implants:

D6010   surgical placement of implant body: endosteal implant

Report 4 times, once per implant body

Abutments:

D6056   prefabricated abutment – includes placement

Report 4 times, once for each implant

D6055   connecting bar – implant supported or abutment supported

In this case the intermediate connection is made of two types of components, the four abutments and one connecting bar. The connecting bar is attached to the abutments and is reported just once, regardless of the number of abutments that support it.

Prosthesis:

D6053   implant/abutment supported removable denture for completely edentulous arch

This code is used for removable complete dentures directly supported by implants or that are directly supported by the individual abutments. When the prosthesis is supported directly by abutments, they usually are custom fabricated with various specialized retentive attachments or devices.

Attachments:

D5862   precision attachment, by report

Coding Exercise #14

A "Maryland" bridge

Melinda was thankful that the accident had not caused more damage. Her face had pretty much recovered from the trauma, but the missing and broken teeth were a constant reminder of that frightful day. Melinda had lost teeth #23 & 24. Tooth #26 was broken and could not be restored. Dr. Trentacosti was reassuring, but when she told Melinda that #26 would have to be extracted, she could tell that Melinda's teeth were pretty important to her.

Dr. Trentacosti discussed implants, which Melinda really liked, but having just started grad school, it would probably be years before she could afford it. When Dr. Trentacosti discussed a "Maryland" bridge, Melinda's eyes lit up. She appreciated that she could preserve her teeth, but still had the option of implants in the future. Dr. Trentacosti proposed a resin bonded porcelain-fused-to-metal (noble) bridge from tooth #22 to #27 with #25 acting as a pier.

How would you code for this Maryland bridge?

Solutions:

The resin bonded or "Maryland" bridge uses the same codes for pontics as a conventional bridge.

The pontic code for teeth #23, 24 & 26 would be:

D6242   pontic – porcelain fused to noble metal

The retainer codes for teeth #22, 25 & 27 are:

D6545   retainer – cast metal for resin bonded fixed prosthesis

Resin bonded bridge retainers (often referred to as wings) are differentiated only by whether they are metal or porcelain. Generally the porcelain/ceramic retainer code (**D6548**) would only be used with a porcelain/ceramic pontic. All cast metal or porcelain fused to metal bridges would utilize the **D6545** code. There is not a code for retainers fabricated out of resin/composite, so **D6999 unspecified fixed prosthodontic procedure, by report** code could be used with a narrative report.

Coding Exercise #15

Temporomandibular joint (TMJ) disorder treatment

Following a comprehensive oral evaluation (**D0150**), Dr. Yonemoto recognized Ms. Mulder's symptoms as a temporomandibular disorder that was of significant complexity. The occasional popping joint and headache had become regular dislocations of the joint, limited opening and nearly constant discomfort. Dr. Yonemoto's evaluation included listening to the joint with a stethoscope, detailed palpation of all the muscles of mastication, recording of occlusal relationships, ranges of motion, and areas of musculoskeletal tenderness.

Ms. Mulder had prepared an extensive health, nutrition and lifestyle history which Dr. Yonemoto now reviewed for TMD risk factors. She identified a number of potential contributing factors to Ms. Mulder's condition. Tooth #18 was missing and tooth #15 had super-erupted to the point that Ms. Mulder could not close without moving her jaw to the right. A tongue thrust habit had left her with a severe anterior open bite.

Dr. Yonemoto decided that following extraction of #15, an orthotic TMJ appliance covering the mandibular occlusal surfaces would allow Ms. Mulder to reposition her jaw to a more comfortable spot and create some anterior occlusal guideplanes. She hoped that after Ms. Mulder was more comfortable, a comprehensive treatment plan could be made.

How would you code Dr. Yonemoto's diagnostic visit?

How could the TMJ appliance be reported to Ms. Mulder's dental insurance?

How would the appliance be reported to a medical plan?

Solutions:

Evaluation:

Due to the limited scope, Dr. Yonemoto can choose one of two problem-focused evaluations:

> **D0140**   **limited oral evaluation – problem focused**
> or;
> **D0160**   **detailed and extensive oral evaluation – problem focused, by report**

In this case, the nature and complexity of the problems suggest that **D0160** would be the most appropriate code for this evaluation. Use of this code requires submission of a narrative report.

Appliance (Dental):

A code for occlusal appliances is found in the Oral & Maxillofacial Surgery category of service:

> **D7880**   **occlusal orthotic device, by report**

This code is used for splints utilized for the treatment of temporomandibular joint dysfunction. It also requires the submission of a descriptive narrative.

Appliance (Medical):

Many dental benefit plans exclude treatment for TMD, so it may be necessary to file a claim using the patient's medical plan. Dentists may file claims with a patient's medical plan as long as he/she is acting within the scope of his/her licensure.

If a claim is filed with a patient's medical plan, it should be reported on a standard medical claim (1500 Health Care Claim) form or filed electronically. Instead of using a procedure from the *Code,* an appropriate CPT®/HCPCS code should be selected to report the procedure. The medical claim form also requires reporting the patient's diagnosis along with the CPT® code for each procedure. The diagnosis codes are known as ICD-9-CM.

For this situation, the CPT®/HCPCS code needed is **HCPCS – S8262 Mandibular orthopedic repositioning device, each.** The ICD-9-CM code for TMJ dysfunction syndrome is **524.60.**

(Continued on following page)

Coding Exercise #15

Solutions:
(Continued)

More information about filing medical benefit plan claims and cross-coding dental to medical services is found in Chapter 10 of *The CDT Companion.*

Super-erupted #15:
Although this tooth could have been treated in a number of ways including, occlusal adjustment, restoration, or endodontic treatment and a crown (various), the code for the extraction is:

> **D7140**   **extraction, erupted tooth or exposed root (elevation and/or forceps removal)**

Quick Quiz #6: Adjusting a TMJ appliance

Q: How do we code for adjusting a TMJ appliance?

A: There is not a specific procedure code to report adjustment of a TMJ appliance. There is a general code for procedures related to treatment of TMJ dysfunctions that could probably be used, **D7899 unspecified TMD therapy, by report.** This code requires that a narrative be included specifying the services that were performed. It could also be used for future appointments for adjustments or other related treatment.

Coding Exercise #16

Sectioning the fixed partial denture of a patient with periodontal disease

Dr. Lopez had been trying to save André's bridge from tooth #13-15 for several years, but the combination of periodontal disease, gingival recession, and now root caries had taken its toll. His latest evaluation left #15 with no hope. André would consider implants, but #15 would have to be extracted and the site allowed to heal before anything else could be done. Dr. Lopez sectioned the bridge distal to #13, extracted #15, refinished and polished the crown on #13 and root planed teeth #12 & 13.

How could these procedures be reported?

Solutions:

A procedure code, effective January 1, 2007, was added to the *Code* to report the sectioning of a bridge when part of the bridge will remain in service after treatment.

D9120   fixed partial denture sectioning
Separation of one or more connections between abutments and/or pontics when some portion of a fixed prosthesis is to remain intact and serviceable following sectioning and extraction or other treatment. Includes all recontouring and polishing of retained portions.

Note that the descriptor says that this code includes recontouring and polishing of the portion of the bridge that will remain intact, but does not include the extraction of any teeth. That procedure is reported using the appropriate extraction code:

D7140   extraction, erupted tooth or exposed root (elevation and/or forceps removal)
Includes routine removal of tooth structure minor smoothing of socket bone, and closure, as necessary.

Scaling of two adjacent teeth in the same quadrant would be coded with:

D4342   periodontal scaling and root planing – one to three teeth per quadrant

Coding Exercise #17

Treating a traumatic wound a mouthguard could have prevented

An eight year old patient arrived at the oral & maxillofacial surgeon's office literally screaming. Mom wasn't much better and Dr. Bennett understood why when he saw the patient; it brought a whole new meaning to the term "game face." Tommy's headfirst slide had resulted in a lower lip full of gravel and a chin raspberry in the making. Dr. Bennett knew things would be better soon, but Tommy was out of control and the cleanup was going to take some time.

An intramuscular injection of 40mg of ketamine provided a reasonable amount of sedation and allowed them to completely debride the wound. Dr. Bennett also placed a couple sutures in the cut in his lip and was looking a lot better. Tommy would make a full recovery, he was lucky not to have broken any teeth.

"Make sure he gets a mouthguard," Dr. Bennett reminded them as they left.

How would you code for Tommy's visit to Dr. Bennett?

What code would Tommy's general dentist use when making him a mouthguard?

Solutions:

Codes that might be used for a parenteral sedative are:

> **D9230**   **inhalation of nitrous oxide /anxiolysis, analgesia**
> or
> **D9248**   **non-intravenous conscious sedation**

Effective January 1, 2007, **D9610 therapeutic drug injection, by report** was revised to exclude the reporting of sedative agents.

There is not a code for traumatic wound debridement, but **D7999 unspecified oral surgery procedure, by report** could be used for that procedure.

Suture placement is reported with a code based on the size of the wound:

> **D7910**   **suture of recent small wounds up to 5cm**

The code for fabrication of an athletic mouthguard is:

> **D9941**   **fabrication of athletic mouthguard**

Quick Quiz #7a: Area of the oral cavity on a claim

Q: When is it necessary to report the area of the oral cavity on a claim?

A: Any procedure that is performed specifically for a limited area of the mouth and for which the nomenclature does not include the area of the oral cavity, the area should be reported. Codes for mouth areas can be found in the CDT manual section that covers tooth numbering and area of the oral cavity.

When a procedure code's nomenclature includes the area of the oral cavity, as in "complete denture – maxillary" it is not necessary to report the area. For "quadrant" codes (e.g., nomenclatures that say "...four or more teeth per quadrant") always report the area of the oral cavity.

Quick Quiz #7b: Tooth numbers for "quadrant" procedures

Q: Should tooth numbers be reported for quadrant or partial quadrant codes?

A: There is no hard-and-fast rule. Generally, when treating specific teeth within a quadrant, tooth numbers should be reported in addition to the quadrant procedure code. In some cases, benefit determination may be accelerated when individual treated teeth are reported.

Quick Quiz #8a: Referred patient consultation

Q: An oral surgery office often gets referrals from other dentists and physicians for patient consultations. Can the surgeon provide other diagnostic services or begin treatment of the patient's problem, if they use the code for consultations (D9310)?

A: Effective January 1, 2007 the consultation code was revised to make it easier to understand.

> D9310 **consultation – diagnostic service provided by dentist or physician other than requesting dentist or physician**
> A patient encounter with a practitioner whose opinion or advice regarding evaluation and/or management of a specific problem; may be requested by another practitioner or appropriate source. The consultation includes an oral evaluation. The consulted practitioner may initiate diagnostic and/or therapeutic services.

You may use this code for your consultation and use other diagnostic and treatment codes when you provide these services, even on the same day.

Quick Quiz #8b: Consultation or problem focused evaluation

Q: When a specialty office receives a referral for consultation should they use the "problem-focused" exam code or the "consultation" code for their first encounter with the patient?

A: Whether to use an evaluation code and which one to use depends on what you do. Many specialty offices use the limited problem-focused exam (**D0140**) when consulting for a specific problem. Whether to use it instead of the consultation code (**D9310**), will depend on the nature and scope of the evaluation and consultation.

Coding Exercise #18

A misbehaving child who needs endodontic treatment and a crown

It was a sad story that Dr. Ashcroft had heard too often. Three year old Melina had Baby Bottle Mouth Syndrome and was waiting in his reception room, crying wildly. Dr. Ashcroft knew she really didn't want to be there, and her pain wasn't helping. They strapped Melina into the papoose board, and she settled down a lot. The tight straps made her feel secure and once the anesthetic had taken effect she stopped crying altogether. Half way through the procedure, Melina fell asleep.

A little later, Melina had three pulpectomies completed and four esthetic-coated stainless steel crowns cemented on her maxillary incisors. After only a little over an hour on the papoose board, Melina was doing great.

How do you document this successful encounter?

Solutions:

A papoose board is a physical restraint that is used for behavior management for young children. There is a generic code for behavior management:

D9920   **behavior management, by report**
May be reported in addition to treatment provided. Should be reported in 15-minute increments.

Behavior management requires a narrative report that describes the method and total time. This procedure is applied in 15 minute units and in this situation it would be reported four times on a claim.

Endodontic procedure:

D3230   **pulpal therapy (resorbable filling)-anterior, primary tooth (excluding final restoration)**

"Pulpal therapy" with a resorbable filling is a typical pulp treatment for primary teeth that have carious pulp exposure. It would be reported three times in this case, once for each tooth.

Primary crowns:

D2934   **prefabricated esthetic coated stainless steel crown – primary tooth**

There are three types of stainless steel crowns for primary teeth: the standard stainless steel crown, one with a resin window and the esthetic coated stainless steel crown. The esthetic coated crown was use in this case and it would be reported four times on the claim.

Coding Exercise #19

Treating a patient suffering from swelling, pain and periodontal disease

Dr. Hart saw a patient for an emergency. The patient was in pain and complained about swelling around one particular tooth. Dr. Hart's emergency evaluation focused on the patient's complaint. She took two periapical films and pocket measurements of the teeth in the area. The swelling was clearly adjacent to tooth #3 and the sulcus gushed a purulent mixture of blood and pus when probed. Dr. Hart treated the patient for a periodontal abscess by gross debridement and draining through the sulcus, irrigating the pocket with Chlorhexidine and prescribing the patient an antibiotic.

How could this encounter be documented?

Solutions:

Since Dr. Hart's evaluation was both problem-focused and limited to the patient's complaint, the appropriate codes for diagnostic procedures would be:

D0140	**limited oral evaluation – problem focused**
D0220	**intraoral – periapical first film**
D0230	**intraoral – periapical each additional film**

Prior to January 1, 2003 there was a procedure code for curettage, which might have been the choice to describe the combination of debridement and drainage, which are generally part of the treatment of a periodontal abscess. That code was deleted by the Code Revision Committee, which agreed with the position taken by the American Academy of Periodontology that intentional curettage has no justifiable application during active treatment for chronic periodontitis. In this case there are a number of codes that might be used to document this service, alone or in combination. Four possible procedure coding options are:

D9110	**palliative (emergency) treatment of dental pain – minor procedure**
	This is typically reported on a "per visit" basis for emergency treatment of dental pain. This code is a "catch-all" code that covers a broad array of procedures.

D7510 incision and drainage of abscess – intraoral soft tissue
Involves incision through mucosa, including periodontal origins.

Discussions at the Code Revision Committee (CRC) meetings indicated that this code was considered by many to be appropriate even when "incision" is made through the gingival sulcus.

D4342 periodontal scaling and root planing – one to three teeth, per quadrant

The descriptor for **D4342** indicates that it is a "definitive procedure," therefore it may not be the appropriate code when the procedure is only managing acute conditions.

D4241 gingival flap procedure, including root planing – one to three contiguous teeth or tooth bounded spaces per quadrant

If a surgical flap is used for open root planing, a gingival flap procedure may be used:

Benefit plan limitations may apply when rendering any of these treatments. For example, some plans do not cover **D9110** at the same appointment with a limited oral evaluation; reporting **D4342** may preclude a benefit for further scaling and root planing procedures in the future, etc. Despite benefit design problems, it is important to code for what was done.

There is not a specific procedure code for irrigation, but the following may be considered:

D4999 unspecified periodontal procedure, by report

Coding Exercise #20 (Part 1)

This exercise encompasses multiple appointments and disciplines related to Periodontics. It addresses some of the "real life" issues that might be encountered as treatment progresses over the course of time, while continuing to highlight some of the principles of coding as they apply particularly to the Periodontics category of the Code. While many offices will not perform all the procedures in this exercise, most of the concepts will be useful in understanding diagnostic, non-surgical and surgical periodontal procedure reporting, as well as the application of several adjunctive procedures.

A partially edentulous patient with bleeding gums, rampant calculus, and white lesions

Dr. Smith pried out Mr. Robinson's lower partial, which had become cemented into place by layers of calculus and months of neglect. What little of the teeth not covered in a mass of calculus was covered with a dark brown veneer of coffee and tobacco residue. Following thirty minutes of hard work with an ultrasonic scaler, the dentist was completing his comprehensive evaluation of the patient that included exploration for caries, evaluation of occlusion, documenting of periodontal probing depths, gingival attachment levels, risk factors for periodontal disease, and a head and neck examination. Dr. Smith noted a white keratinized patch in the left retromolar pad area. He noted from Mr. Robinson's health history, that the patient was taking medication for Type II diabetes, that he smoked, and that his chief complaint was "bleeding gums."

Dr. Smith took radiographs of the entire lower arch including four posterior and two anterior periapicals as well as two bitewings on the left and one on the right side. The evaluation indicated that Mr. Robinson had a full upper denture and lower removable partial denture. He was missing #17, 19, 21, 23, 24, 25, 26, 30, 31 & 32. Bone loss around the remaining teeth ranged from 1-4 mm and subgingival calculus was still present. Pocket depths were all measured at 4-7 mm, and there was Class II furcation involvement of #18. The gingiva exhibited generalized moderate hyperemia and was dark red in color indicating chronic inflammation, but Dr. Smith expected that the fiery red outline of Mr. Robinson's partial would fade significantly before the next appointment, assuming that he took the denture out to clean it between now and then.

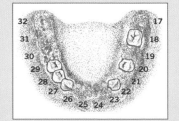

Today's treatment included:
- Gross removal of calculus and stain
- Complete evaluation (exam)
- Radiographs (6 PA & 3 BW)
- Disaggregated transepithelial biopsy (brush) of white patch
- Dispense one 16 oz. bottle of Chlorhexidine Gluconate rinse

How would you code for this appointment?

Solutions:

Today's Appointment:

D4355   **full mouth debridement to enable comprehensive evaluation and diagnosis**
The gross removal of plaque and calculus that interfere with the ability of the dentist to perform a comprehensive oral evaluation. This preliminary procedure does not preclude the need for additional procedures.

This procedure is done prior to completing diagnosis when it is not possible to adequately access tooth surfaces and periodontal areas because of excessive plaque and calculus. Although the descriptor for this code indicates that other procedures may be necessary, payers may have policies that disallow this procedure on the same day as evaluations or prophylaxis.

D0150   **comprehensive oral evaluation – new or established patient**
or
D0180   **comprehensive periodontal evaluation – new or established patient**

In this case either comprehensive evaluation code would be acceptable. The only difference between the codes is the requirement that the patient have signs or symptoms of periodontal disease for **D0180.** Both codes may be used by general dentists and specialists.

The periapical and bitewing radiographs do not match the full mouth series definition that was added as the D0210 intraoral – complete series..." procedure code effective January 1. 2009. Therefore the radiographs in this scenario would be reported using the periapical and bitewing codes:

D0220   **intraoral – periapical first film**

D0230   **intraoral – periapical each additional film**

(Report five times, one entry for each additional film)

D0273   **bitewings – three films**

(Note: **D0273** was removed from the Code in 1985 but was returned to the Code in 2007.)

D7288   **brush biopsy – transepithelial sample collection**

The brush biopsy samples disaggregated dermal and epithelial cells. A positive sample usually requires follow-up with an architecturally intact incisional or excisional sample. The code to use when dispensing Chlorhexidine Gluconate is:

D9630   **other drugs and/or medicaments, by report**

This code requires a narrative report, which usually includes the drug, quantity, and reason for using that medicine.

Coding Exercise #20 (Part 2)

A periodontally compromised patient with a tobacco habit

The focus of Mr. Robinson's treatment would be his periodontal disease and managing risk factors. Dr. Smith knew that non-surgical treatment would only go so far with Mr. Robinson's problems, but he also knew that Mr. Robinson was not a good candidate for surgery at this time. He recommended a conservative approach while Mr. Robinson addressed his other health issues. His treatment plan was:

Second Appointment:

- Discussion of the risks of tobacco use and contributory habits, design of a program to quit, along with a prescription for "The Patch"

- Scaling and root planing of the entire lower right quadrant using a non-injectable periodontal gel in the sulcus for anesthesia, followed by irrigation of each sulcus with Chlorhexidine Gluconate rinse.

Third Appointment:

- Review of progress on tobacco use cessation program and results of biopsy.

- Scaling and root planing of the entire lower left quadrant using mandibular block anesthesia, followed by placement of an antibacterial gel (Atridox®) in each sulcus.

How would you code for each appointment?

Solutions:

Second Appointment:

D1320   **tobacco counseling for the control and prevention of oral disease**
Tobacco prevention and cessation services reduce patient risks of developing tobacco-related oral diseases and conditions and improves prognosis for certain dental therapies.

D4342   **periodontal scaling and root planing – one to three teeth per quadrant**

A separate code is available in the adjunctive services category of the *Code* that may be used when a dentist wants to document and separately report delivery of local anesthesia:

D9215   **local anesthesia in conjunction with operative or surgical procedures**

Not all dental benefit plans provide separate reimbursement of local anesthesia.

No code exists for sulcular irrigation. **D4999** (unspecified periodontal procedure, by report) might be used on a "by report" basis.

Third Appointment:

D1320   **(tobacco counseling for the control and prevention of oral disease)**

Dr. Smith may elect to use this code again for a second appointment. The *Code* does not indicate that D1320 as a single use procedure, but payers, either dental or medical, might consider it that way.

D4342   **periodontal scaling and root planing – one to three teeth per quadrant**

Although there are two tooth bounded spaces in this quadrant, the codes for root planing count only the number of teeth actually treated in determining the correct code.

The placement of Atridox® (or other medicaments like Arrestin®, Actisite® or the Periochip®) is coded using:

D4381   **localized delivery of antimicrobial agents via a controlled release vehicle into diseased crevicular tissue, per tooth, by report**

This code is appropriate for these medicines because they utilize a controlled release mechanism. This would exclude passive delivery mechanisms like irrigation. It should be noted that some carriers will pay this on the same date of service as a **D4341** or **D4342** only if the pocket depth is sufficient to hold the medicament. (4.5-5mm minimum). Others will only pay **D4381** after 10 to 14 days post-scaling and root planing. The theory being that one should wait to see if the scaling & root planing alone will produce sufficient shrinkage to render the antibiotic usage unnecessary.

Coding Exercise #20 (Part 3)

A patient with persistent 5mm pockets and bone loss

A year later, Mr. Robinson was a new man. He had successfully quit smoking for more than nine months and no longer had to take medication for diabetes, which was now less severe and easily managed with a normal diet. His oral hygiene was good and the gingiva had a much healthier appearance, although there was some persistent 5-6 mm pocketing and bleeding on probing. Dr. Smith had noted his steady improvement at each periodontal maintenance appointment. The white patch, which had been diagnosed as leukoplakia, was now almost entirely gone.

Dr. Smith praised Mr. Robinson for his success at reducing his risk factors and decided that his condition now warranted further treatment of his periodontal disease with surgery.

This is the treatment plan Dr. Smith recommended:

Appointment one:

- Modified Widman surgery and open root debridement and planing of the lower right quadrant

Appointment two:

- Osseous surgery of the lower left quadrant, with placement of a freeze-dried bone graft and placement of a resorbable barrier membrane in the buccal furcation of #19

How would you code each of these procedures?

Solutions:

Appointment one:

D4241 **gingival flap procedure, including root planing – one to three contiguous teeth or tooth bounded spaces per quadrant**

The modified Widman procedure is a non-osseous periodontal surgery that includes root planing. This quadrant has several missing teeth and teeth spaces, but none of the spaces are bounded (teeth on either side) within this quadrant. This leaves just the three contiguous teeth (#27, 28, and 29) for this flap procedure.

Appointment two:

D4260 **osseous surgery (including flap entry and closure) – four or more contiguous teeth or tooth bounded spaces per quadrant**

Even though there are only three teeth in this quadrant, there are two bounded teeth spaces (#19, 21) in this quadrant. Because these teeth and bounded teeth spaces are contiguous (next to each other), there are a total of five, which makes **D4260** the appropriate code.

D4263 **bone replacement graft – first site in quadrant**

D4266 **guided tissue regeneration – resorbable barrier; per site**

These services are coded in addition to the osseous surgery and are reported based on the number of sites.

From the *Code:*

Site: A term used to describe a single area, position, or locus. The word "site" is frequently used to indicate an area of soft tissue recession on a single tooth or an osseous defect adjacent to a single tooth; also used to indicate soft tissue defects and/or osseous defects in edentulous tooth positions.
- If two contiguous teeth have areas of soft tissue recession, each area of recession is a single site.
- If two contiguous teeth have adjacent but separate osseous defects, each defect is a single site.
- If two contiguous teeth have a communicating interproximal osseous defect, it should be considered a single site.
- All non-communicating osseous defects are single sites.
- All edentulous non-contiguous tooth positions are single sites.
- Depending on the dimensions of the defect, up to two contiguous edentulous tooth positions may be considered a single site.

Quick Quiz #9: Scaling and root planing, and prophylaxis – same patient, same day

Q: During a routine prophylaxis, isolated areas of pocketing are detected. It is determined that scaling and root planing is needed for two teeth in a single quadrant. Can you report both the code for prophylaxis and root planing (D1110 and D4342) on the same day?

A: There are no restrictions in either scaling and root planing code (partial or full quadrant) or the prophylaxis codes that would preclude their use with any other procedure codes.

Some third-party plans may have policies that preclude paying a benefit for both of these procedures on the same date of service.

Which biopsy code should I use?

There are three codes typically used for soft tissue biopsies, which differentiate the techniques based on the depth and structural integrity of the tissue sample.

D7286   **biopsy of oral tissue – soft tissue**
For surgical removal of an architecturally intact specimen only. This code is not used at the same time as codes for apicoectomy/periradicular curettage.

D7287   **exfoliative cytological sample collection**
For collection of non-transepithelial cytology sample via mild scraping of the oral mucosa.

D7288   **brush biopsy – transepithelial sample collection**
For collection of oral disaggregated transepithelial cells via rotational brushing of the oral mucosa.

Codes **D7287** and **D7288** are used for cell sampling biopsies that do not maintain tissue architecture, depending on the depth and method of sampling. Code **D7286** would be used for incisional and excisional tissue samples that maintain the original structure.

Coding Exercise #21

When a "quadrant" procedure involves teeth that cross the midline

Lars was pretty good about taking care of his teeth, but struggled with his gums because of an anti-seizure medicine that he took for epilepsy. A hockey accident as a 25-year-old had left him with a fixed bridge from #22-27, replacing #'s 23, 24, 25, & 26. Although he brushed and flossed diligently, he had a hard time with flossing under the bridge because gum tissue had grown up around it. This seemed to make his gum problem even worse.

Now Lars had 4-5 mm pocket measurements around #22 & #27 because of the heavy fibrotic tissue. There was no apparent loss of bone around these teeth, so Dr. Svenson recommended surgically removing the excess tissue and restoring a more cleansable gingival contour around Lars' bridge.

How would you code this visit?

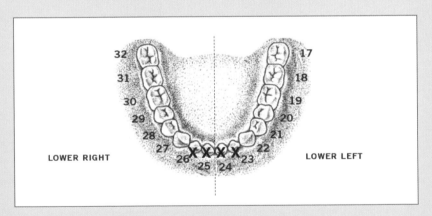

Solutions:

Dr. Svenson's reshaping of Lars' gingival tissue would be coded as:

D4211 **gingivectomy or gingivoplasty – one to three contiguous teeth or tooth bounded spaces per quadrant**

The code would be used twice, once for each quadrant. Even though the two teeth being treated are contiguous with the bounded space between them, the teeth are in different quadrants and the space is not bounded in either quadrant.

This procedure would usually be reported by listing the tooth numbers of the teeth treated. When reporting "quadrant" codes listing both tooth numbers and quadrants may facilitate third-party payer claim adjudication.

Coding Exercise #22

Treating acute pulpitis

Vincent called the office begging the receptionist to be seen today. When he arrived with a cup of ice water, Dr. Stevenson had pretty much made his diagnosis of acute pulpitis, without even looking at the tooth. He opened #5 to gain access to the pulp chamber and removed the tissue with a broach. He closed the tooth with a temporary filling.

Ten days later Vincent returned to have the root canal completed. The canal was opened, thoroughly flushed and cleaned, then obturated with gutta percha and an appropriate sealer.

How would you code for the endodontic treatment on each appointment?

Solutions:

Appointment 1:

> **D3221**   **pulpal debridement**
>
> **D2940**   **protective restoration**

These procedures describe the simple removal of acutely inflamed pulp tissue, and closure with a temporary restoration, for the relief of pain. This is not a definitive endodontic treatment.

Appointment 2:

> **D3320**   **endodontic therapy, bicuspid tooth (excluding final restoration)**

This is a completed root canal therapy using an appropriate endodontic therapy procedure code.

Language in the descriptor of **D3221 pulpal debridement** precludes the same provider from reporting this procedure on the same date as an endodontic procedure. Since the date of completion of the root canal is different from the date of initiation of the procedure, and the patient presented with an emergency, both codes may be reported.

Coding Exercise #23

Reporting a multi appointment endodontic therapy service

Vincent had been having a toothache off and on for several weeks. He knew that it was the tooth Dr. Stevenson had been recommending for a root canal at his last visit. When he called the office he was eager to get an appointment.

Given the choice of seeing Dr. Stevenson for an emergency visit today or scheduling for definitive treatment two days later, he opted for the treatment appointment, figuring that he would be OK on ibuprofen for another two days. When Dr. Stevenson opened tooth #5 it flowed with a bloody fluid drainage.

After thorough instrumentation and flushing with sodium hypochlorite solution, the pulp chamber was cleaned and shaped, but Dr. Stevenson was unable to get the canal dry enough to obturate, since there was a persistent weepy flow. The canal was medicated with a calcium hydroxide paste and closed with a temporary cement.

Ten days later Vincent returned to have the root canal completed. The canal was opened, thoroughly flushed and cleaned. Obturation with gutta percha and an appropriate sealer was now possible because there was no longer fluid drainage.

How would you code for the endodontic treatment on each appointment?

What if when Vincent returned it was determined that the root canal could not be completed because a vertical crack in the root was preventing the apical infection from resolving?

Solutions:

Appointment 1:

> **D3320**   **endodontic therapy, bicuspid tooth (excluding final restoration)**

Appointment 2:

No codes, but claim should be submitted upon completion of endodontic procedure.

This is a two appointment root canal. The patient had pain, but not enough to come in as an emergency. Since the initial appointment was scheduled, it would not be appropriate to code the initial treatment as a **D3221 pulpal debridement.**

Fractured root:
Since the root canal could not be completed Dr. Stevenson should use:

> **D3332**   **incomplete endodontic therapy; inoperable, unrestorable or fractured tooth**

in place of endodontic treatment code **D3320**.

What if there is no code describing a procedure?

When there is no applicable procedure code, use the "unspecified... procedure, by report" (Dnn99) procedure codes.

The "unspecified...procedure, by report" codes are for those situations where, in the opinion of the dentist, none of the codes contained in the *Code on Dental Procedures and Nomenclature* accurately describe the services provided to the patient. These "unspecified...procedure, by report" codes (e.g., **D2999 unspecified restorative procedure, by report**) are included for each category of dental services, with the exception of Preventive. A third-party payer may request additional documentation of certain procedures regardless of the presence of the narrative "report."

When you submit a narrative, describe the procedure performed. If applicable, include the necessity for extra time, use of new technology, etc. Include supplementary information that you feel will be helpful in determining benefits, or which is required by the third-party payer.

If a multi-page narrative is submitted on paper, include the patient's name on each page and staple all pages together.

Quick Quiz #10: A procedure involving teeth in a sextant

Q: How would you report procedures that involve a sextant? For example, if a doctor performs an alveoloplasty for teeth #6 through #11:

A: Treatment in one of the posterior sextants must be coded using the corresponding quadrant code based on the number of teeth (or spaces) involved. When teeth in two quadrants but the same anterior sextant are treated, as in the example, it is necessary to use the quadrant code referring to "1 to 3 teeth (or spaces)" twice.

Although there are area codes for each of the six sextants printed in the CDT manual section on tooth numbering and areas of the oral cavity, all references to sextants have been removed from the *Code*. Please note too that sextant codes are not permitted in a HIPAA compliant electronic transaction.

Coding Exercise #24

D4910 v. D1110 on recall visits after periodontal therapy

During a recent study club meeting Dr. Croseus, a general dentist, asked aloud "After active periodontal therapy and a period of maintenance is it ever appropriate for a patient to receive a prophylaxis procedure in lieu of a periodontal maintenance procedure during a recall visit?"

Dr. Abraxis, another member of the study club, asked for clarification, "Are you talking about alternating procedures performed so that both periodontal maintenance and prophylaxis can be done on a continuing basis?" The answer was yes.

Dr. Croseus was also concerned with the mantra "Once a perio patient, always a perio patient" that appears to limit a dentist's decision-making when assessing a patient's clinical condition. Dr. Abraxis chimed in. "Treatment planning and decisions on what procedure to deliver on a certain day are a matter of clinical judgment by the treating dentist. A dental benefit plan covers some portion of the cost for necessary dental care, not what services a dentist may or may not deliver to a patient."

What then are the options?

1. Follow-up patients who have received active periodontal therapy (surgical or non-surgical) can receive the periodontal maintenance service described in **D4910 periodontal maintenance.** A periodontal maintenance procedure includes removal of plaque, calculus and site specific scaling and root planing and follows periodontal therapy.

2. If the treating dentist determines that a patient's periodontal health can be augmented with a periodic routine prophylaxis, delivery of this service and reporting with code **D1110 prophylaxis – adult** would be appropriate. A prophylaxis procedure includes removal of plaque, calculus and stains and is intended to control local irritational factors.

Dr. Abraxis concluded by stating, "If in the dentist's professional judgment a patient can benefit from periodic prophylaxis in addition to periodontal maintenance procedures, for instance to control irritational factors, then those services should be performed. There is nothing in the D1110 and D4910 nomenclatures or descriptors that say these procedures are mutually exclusive."

Coding Exercise #25

Preventive Resin Restorations

The patient arrived at the office for a recall visit. On the previous recall visit six months ago, Dr. Sucrose noted that this patient had nutritional counseling as well as several teeth that needed to be restored due to decay.

Before doing anything Dr. Sucrose decided that a caries risk assessment should be completed, using the form posted on ADA.org. A look at the answers on the form – especially the combination of frequent consumption of soft drinks and energy drinks, past interproximal restorations, and two incipient carious lesions – led to the conclusion that the patient is at moderate risk of continuing caries development.

During the oral exam the doctor did indeed see what appeared to be small carious lesions on the occlusal surfaces of #s 30 and 31. After limited excavation, the cavitated lesions ended up confined within enamel only and never extended into the dentin.

Dr. Sucrose concluded that a minimally invasive restorative technique would be able to restore the tooth structure damaged by caries, and prevent progression of the disease into the dentin. A composite resin would be used to restore tooth form and function along with an unfilled resin used afterwards to seal out all the radiating grooves.

What then is the appropriate code to document this procedure? Dr. Sucrose knew that D2391 (one surface posterior composite) is not appropriate since the dentin was untouched. Likewise, D1351 (sealant – per tooth) isn't applicable since decay was present.

Solutions:

D1352 **preventive resin restoration in a moderate to high caries risk patient – permanent tooth**

This entry was added to the *Code on Dental Procedures and Nomenclature* effective January 1, 2011. It was added to enable documentation of a conservative restorative procedure where caries, erosion or other conditions affect the natural form and function of the tooth. This procedure is part of many dental school curricula under names that vary by school and region (e.g., preventive resin restoration; conservative resin restoration; minimally invasive resin restoration).

Caries risk assessment information, including the evaluation forms, is available on line at – http://www.ada.org/2752.aspx?currentTab=2

Coding Exercise #26

Coronectomy

It was Friday the 13th and Dr. Moulage, an oral and maxillofacial surgeon, had just completed consultations with two patients referred by their general dentists, who both faced similar complications.

Patient 1 –
A 38 year old male presents with chronic pericornitis associated with a deep mesio-angular impaction of tooth # 32. There is gingival inflammation and substantial bone loss surrounding the crown. The root of the tooth extends well past the inferior alveolar nerve canal and it is the dentist's opinion that removal of the entire tooth is a substantial risk to the nerve.

Patient 2 –
A 19 year old female presents for evaluation and treatment of a dentigerous cyst, associated with an impacted supernumerary tooth in the area of #20, displaced inferiorly and is encroaching on the left mental foramen. After evaluation and examination, the dentist determines that total removal of the supernumerary tooth risks injury to the Inferior Alveolar Nerve.

What procedure codes would be used to document the services delivered and planned?

Solutions:

Each patient's record would have the same procedure codes.

For today's consultation –

D9310 **consultation – diagnostic service provided by dentist or physician other than requesting dentist or physician**

For the planned procedure –

D7251 **coronectomy – intentional partial tooth removal**

D7251 was added to the *Code on Dental Procedures and Nomenclature* effective January 1, 2011. It was added to enable documentation of intentional partial tooth removal that is performed when a neurovascular complication is likely if the entire impacted tooth is removed. The procedure avoids complications involving the Inferior Alveolar Nerve and the Lingual Nerve.

Coding Exercise #27

Harvesting Bone

Two years following an ATV accident the patient was still dealing with the after effects of the comminuted fracture of his anterior maxilla. A traumatic defect and oro-nasal fistula, not much different from a congenital alveolar cleft, still existed.

Dr. Huey, his oral surgeon, recommended closure of the fistula and reconstruction of the bony deficit prior to prosthetic reconstruction. The doctor planned to do this as an in office procedure utilizing an autogenous bone graft from the tibia.

What codes would be used to document these procedures?

Solutions:

Two codes would be used to document the services Dr. Huey planned to do in the office. The grafting procedure code is:

D7955 **repair of maxillofacial soft tissue and/or hard tissue defect**
Reconstruction of surgical, traumatic, or congenital defects of the facial bones, including the mandible, may utilize autograft, allograft, or alloplastic materials in conjunction with soft tissue procedures to repair and restore the facial bones to form and function. This does not include obtaining the graft...

Fortunately for Dr. Huey the grafting procedure occurred after January 1, 2011. On that date a new code was effective that provided a means to report the separate procedure for obtaining osseous material for the purpose of grafting to a distant site. The harvesting code is:

D7295 **harvest of bone for use in autogenous grafting procedure**
Reported in addition to those autogenous graft placement procedures that do not include harvesting of bone.

This entry was added to enable documentation of the harvesting procedure when the grafting procedure (e.g., D4263; D7953; D7955) does not include obtaining bone to be grafted.

Revising the *Code* 6

CDT
Companion

Chapter 6
Revising the *Code*

The Code on Dental Procedures and Nomenclature is maintained by the ADA's Code Revision Committee (CRC), which was formed in 2001 and represents an equal balance of interests between the ADA and the Payer sector of the dental community. The CRC's voting membership is comprised of six payer representatives, one each from America's Health Insurance Plans (AHIP), the Blue Cross Blue Shield Association (BCBSA), the Centers for Medicare and Medicaid Services (CMS), Delta Dental Plans Association (DDPA), National Association of Dental Plans (NADP), and a National Purchaser of Dental Benefits. For the dental profession there are six representatives from the ADA's Council on Dental Benefit Programs (CDBP).

Code review and revision is a dynamic process that results in changes that reflect evolution in clinical dentistry. Revisions to the *Code* are published and effective biennially, at the start of odd-numbered years. In addition to the scheduled CRC meetings and CRC conference calls, the ADA's representatives engage in their own review and evaluation of each requested change to the *Code* before every CRC meeting.

The ADA, as the CRC's Secretariat, provides staff support to the review and revision process. Please visit the ADA's Web site (www.ada.org/goto/dentalcode) for more information about:

- The overall process and its schedule

- Change request forms and submission

- Inventories of requests, including the specific requested action, to be addressed during a CRC meeting

- Summary reports of actions taken on requested changes to the *Code*, including rationales for the decision to decline a change request

Any changes accepted in the next revision process will be included in the version of the *Code* published in *CDT 2013/2014* that is scheduled to be released in the fall of 2012.

Requests for Changes to the *Code*

The *Code* can be changed for many reasons. These can include changes in technology or materials that have led to new procedures not currently described in the *Code*; or it may be necessary to improve clarity and accuracy of nomenclature and descriptors; or it may be necessary to delete obsolete codes.

Changes are submitted by individual dentists and their staffs, study clubs, specialty groups, dental manufacturing and technology companies or third-party payers. Anyone may submit a code change request.

Submission guidelines, criteria, instructions and the appropriate submission form can be downloaded at www.ada.org/goto/dentalcode. The submission form is a Microsoft Word® document that is intended to be completed and saved at your office, and transmitted to the ADA via email to *dentalcode@ada.org*. For assistance please contact the ADA Member Service Center – Members may use the toll free number on the ADA membership card; non-members can call 312-440-2500.

An idea becomes a new procedure code

In 2004, as a response to concerns about providing adequate access to care for toddlers and infants, the ADA Board of Trustees adopted the following resolution:

> **B-63-2004. Resolved,** that the Council on Dental Benefit Programs, through the Code Revision Committee, develop a code in the ADA *Code on Dental Procedures and Nomenclature* for an oral examination and consultation for a patient under three years of age.

Later that year, it was adopted as a policy by the ADA House of Delegates. During 2005, ADA Council on Dental Benefit Programs (CDBP) staff and volunteers researched and proposed suitable language for a new code. Concurrently, the American Academy of Pediatric Dentistry (AAPD) submitted a new code request for a similar procedure. In September 2005 the CDBP submitted a new code request to the Code Revision Committee (CRC) for consideration. At the final meeting of the revision cycle in February 2006, after consultation with AAPD, the CRC amended and adopted the request that became code:

D0145   **oral evaluation for a patient under three years of age and counseling with primary caregiver**

D0145 became effective on January 1, 2007. This is just one way that an idea can become a new procedure code.

Dental Claim Submission

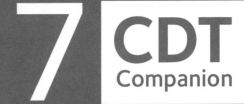

Chapter 7
Dental Claim Submission

ADA Dental Claim Form Updates

As of 2000, the number of dentists submitting claims electronically was nearly 42%. This percentage is increasing annually at the rate of a little over 4.5% per year, according to information compiled by the American Dental Association. Depending on the dental benefit plans your office works with and your individual methodologies, your numbers may vary. The ADA's paper claim form was last updated effective January 1, 2007 to enable reporting of the HIPAA National Provider Identifier (NPI). This updated version may prompt some changes to your software programs if you print paper claim forms.

You will find complete, detailed instructions of the claim form in the current CDT manual. *(A sample copy of the claim form and instructions follows later in this chapter, see p.122)*

There are some fields of information that are not present on prior versions of the ADA claim form. Fields of information found in the current claim form (2006©American Dental Association) are used in the electronic format as well. For those using older versions of the paper claim form, it is important to understand how these newer fields are to be completed when preparing to use the current form.

Transition from Paper Forms to Electronic Data Interchange (EDI)

Electronic Data Interchange (EDI) is the electronic transfer of information between two computer systems using a standard format. Data is exchanged using the electronic equivalents of standard business documents. EDI has been widespread in the banking and retail industries and is fast becoming a mainstay in the health care industry for everything from benefits eligibility to dental claims, claim status, through reimbursements.

Federal regulations arising from HIPAA (see *Chapter 11 - HIPAA Overview*) specify the health care EDI transactions that would be used by dentists.

Parts of an EDI Transaction

A standard EDI electronic document, or transaction set, is made up of data segments. Each data segment contains different types of information with each segment containing data elements. You can think of data elements as words that, for example, describe particular things such as patient name and address, dental procedure(s), or units of measure. These "words" are combined into different data segments that are analogous to paragraphs, with separate paragraphs to contain information about the patient, the services rendered, the insurance company, etc.

In addition, an EDI transaction set has three parts: a header, a main body or detail area, and a trailer. An electronic claim would, for example, have a header that contains control information (e.g., who is sending the transaction and who is to receive it). Itemized information, what is contained in the data segments, is in the main body or detail area. The trailer identifies the individual (e.g., one patient's claim) transaction's end and includes technical information that the recipient needs to be sure that all the transmitted data (e.g., data content segments) have been received for processing.

Data transmitted using EDI does not have to be re-keyed thereby eliminating additional data entry errors and the cost of data entry staff. Complete transaction sets are usually not transmitted individually. They would be accumulated as generated and sorted in batches according to the destination (e.g., by third party payer). Each destination group is packaged together and transmitted as a single unit. This electronic process mirrors what happens with letters and other paper correspondence that is sent via the US Postal Service or a special overnight delivery company.

Submitting Dental Claims Electronically

Dentists submitting claims electronically must do so using the HIPAA standard dental claim (ANSI ASC X12N Transaction Set 837 for dental claims). These electronic transactions may be transmitted in a variety of ways, including:

1. **Submit claims through an intermediary vendor to a payer.** Dentists who have practice management software with a billing component may use a vendor such as a billing entity or clearinghouse to transmit dental claims to payers. Such a vendor is a company that is contracted by the dental office to complete and submit claims for the dental practice, which means that the dentist does not have to be concerned with establishing and maintaining a separate electronic connection with each payer. A billing entity may provide additional services such as verifying information and ensuring that all necessary fields on the claim have been completed.

2. **Submit claims directly to the payer.** Dentists submitting claims directly to payers must have an appropriate secure and tested connection with each payer. When submitting claims electronically, extra fields beyond the standard fields of the ADA Dental Claim Form may need to be completed for each claim. Although HIPAA has standardized claims transactions, various data elements are situational and may not be required. Due to the complexity and specific nature of each payer's claims submission processes, many dental practices employ staff solely dedicated to the submission of claims and payment recovery.

3. **Securely transmit claims over the Internet.** This method eliminates the need for separate electronic connections to individual payers. EDI typically focuses on large batch claims, whereas the Internet is used primarily for single transactions with rapid response. Internet connectivity may enable dental practices to convey patient information to verify benefit eligibility, as well as for claim submission

Currently, EDI is the primary method used for claims submission. However, the inability of some claims submission systems to become HIPAA compliant may cause a shift to an Application Service Provider (ASP) or an Internet enabled or browser based model for claims submission. An ASP hosts its own or a third-party's software and hardware that a dentist may use without having to purchase or install the software and hardware in the practice. ASPs can provide services like a clearinghouse, and may charge the dentist a monthly usage fee, a per-transaction charge, or both.

National Provider Identifier (NPI)

The National Provider Identifier (NPI) is a federal requirement for all HIPAA-covered dentists, e.g., those sending claims electronically. An NPI is a unique, government-issued, standard identification number for individual health care providers and provider organizations like clinics, hospitals, schools and group practices. The government has contracted with an external company for processing applications and developing these random 10-digit numbers for applicants. Applications to obtain an NPI began on May 23, 2005.

When the NPI regulation was published in 2005 the federal government expected that its use would spread beyond HIPAA standard transactions. Dentists may be subject to state level regulations (e.g., Minnesota) and participating provider contracts with third-party payers that require use of NPI on paper claims.

NPI information is posted on the ADA Web page at www.ada.org/goto/npi. Please refer to that Web site for current information. NPI questions, comments or concerns may be conveyed to ADA staff via e-mail to *NPI@ada.org.*

As of May 23, 2007 anyone who used standard electronic transactions (electronic claims, eligibility verifications, claims status inquiries, etc.) was required by federal law to include NPIs on these transactions. In addition, those dentists who use only paper, voice or "fax" to transmit these communications may find NPIs useful. The ADA encourages all dentists to apply for NPIs as an NPI has some advantages over identifiers now in use:

- Once implemented across the health care industry, the NPI will be accepted by all dental plans as a valid provider identifier on electronic dental claims and other standard electronic transactions.

- Dentists will not have to maintain multiple, arbitrary identifiers required by dental plans, nor will they have to remember which number to use with which dental plan.

- Introduces an important element of standardization to electronic transactions that should improve transaction acceptance rates.

However, the NPI does not do any of the following:

- Replace the DEA number when required for prescribing controlled substances or other DEA-regulated activities.

- Replace state-issued licenses and certifications verifying a provider's licensing or qualifications.

- Replace Social Security Number, individual Tax ID, or Employer ID for tax purposes.

How to Apply for an NPI

Applying for an NPI is free and relatively easy: Visit https://nppes.cms.hhs.gov/ NPPES/Welcome.do and read the instructions carefully, complete the questionnaire and submit your application. This should take about 20-30 minutes. After confirmation of your data's receipt, you should receive your NPI via e-mail in one to five business days. A downloadable application form is also available. Download the application form, print, complete and mail per the instructions. The NPPES does not accept faxed applications. Processing of paper applications takes about 20 business days.

There are two types of NPI available to dentists and dental practices:

Type 1. Individual Provider – All individual dentists are eligible to apply for Type 1 NPIs, regardless of whether they are covered by HIPAA.

Type 2. Organization Provider – A health care provider that is an organization, such as a group practice or corporation. Individual dentists who are incorporated may enumerate as Type 2 providers, in addition to being enumerated as a Type 1. All incorporated dental practices and group practices are eligible for enumeration as type 2 providers.

On paper, there is no way to distinguish a Type 1 from a Type 2 in the absence of any associated data; they are identical in format. Additional information on NPI and enumeration can be obtained from the ADA's Web site: www.ada.org/goto/npi.

ADA Claim Form

The Dental Claim Form has evolved to keep practice with current treatment modalities and reporting requirements. This is a copy of the current form and instructions.

American Dental Association Dental Claim Form

HEADER INFORMATION

1. Type of Transaction (Mark all applicable boxes)
   - [ ] Statement of Actual Services
   - [ ] Request for Predetermination/Preauthorization
   - [ ] EPSDT/Title XIX

2. Predetermination/Preauthorization Number

INSURANCE COMPANY/DENTAL BENEFIT PLAN INFORMATION

3. Company/Plan Name, Address, City, State, Zip Code

OTHER COVERAGE

4. Other Dental or Medical Coverage?   [ ] No (Skip 5-11)   [ ] Yes (Complete 5-11)

5. Name of Policyholder/Subscriber in #4 (Last, First, Middle Initial, Suffix)

6. Date of Birth (MM/DD/CCYY)

7. Gender   [ ] M [ ] F

8. Policyholder/Subscriber ID

9. Plan/Group Number

10. Patient's Relationship to Person Named in #5   [ ] Self [ ] Spouse [ ] Dependent [ ] Other

11. Other Insurance Company/Dental Benefit Plan Name, Address, City, State, Zip Code

POLICYHOLDER/SUBSCRIBER INFORMATION (For Insurance Company Named in #3)

12. Policyholder/Subscriber Name (Last, First, Middle Initial, Suffix), Address, City, State, Zip Code

13. Date of Birth (MM/DD/CCYY)

14. Gender   [ ] M [ ] F

15. Policyholder/Subscriber ID

16. Plan/Group Number

17. Employer Name

PATIENT INFORMATION

18. Relationship to Policyholder/Subscriber in #12 Above   [ ] Self [ ] Spouse [ ] Dependent Child [ ] Other

19. Student Status   [ ] FTS [ ] PTS

20. Name (Last, First, Middle Initial, Suffix), Address, City, State, Zip Code

21. Date of Birth (MM/DD/CCYY)

22. Gender   [ ] M [ ] F

23. Patient ID/Account # (Assigned by Dentist)

RECORD OF SERVICES PROVIDED

	24. Procedure Date (MM/DD/CCYY)	25. Area of Oral Cavity	26. Tooth System	27. Tooth Number(s) or Letter(s)	28. Tooth Surface	29. Procedure Code	30. Description	31. Fee
1								
2								
3								
4								
5								
6								
7								
8								
9								
10								

MISSING TEETH INFORMATION

34. (Place an "X" on each missing tooth)

Permanent: 1 2 3 4 5 6 7 8 9 10 11 12 13 14 15 16 / 32 31 30 29 28 27 26 25 24 23 22 21 20 19 18 17

Primary: A B C D E F G H I J / T S R Q P O N M L K

32. Other Fee(s)

33. Total Fee

35. Remarks

AUTHORIZATIONS

36. I have been informed of the treatment plan and associated fees. I agree to be responsible for all charges for dental services and materials not paid by my dental benefit plan, unless prohibited by law, or the treating dentist or dental practice has a contractual agreement with my plan prohibiting all or a portion of such charges. To the extent permitted by law, I consent to your use and disclosure of my protected health information to carry out payment activities in connection with this claim.

X _____
Patient/Guardian signature   Date

37. I hereby authorize and direct payment of the dental benefits otherwise payable to me, directly to the below named dentist or dental entity.

X _____
Subscriber signature   Date

BILLING DENTIST OR DENTAL ENTITY (Leave blank if dentist or dental entity is not submitting claim on behalf of the patient or insured/subscriber)

48. Name, Address, City, State, Zip Code

49. NPI

50. License Number

51. SSN or TIN

52. Phone Number ( ) –

52A. Additional Provider ID

ANCILLARY CLAIM/TREATMENT INFORMATION

38. Place of Treatment   [ ] Provider's Office [ ] Hospital [ ] ECF [ ] Other

39. Number of Enclosures (00 to 99)   Radiograph(s) Oral Image(s) Model(s)

40. Is Treatment for Orthodontics?   [ ] No (Skip 41-42)   [ ] Yes (Complete 41-42)

41. Date Appliance Placed (MM/DD/CCYY)

42. Months of Treatment

43. Replacement of Prosthesis?   [ ] No [ ] Yes (Complete 44)

44. Date of Prior Placement (MM/DD/CCYY)

45. Treatment Resulting from   [ ] Occupational illness/injury [ ] Auto accident [ ] Other accident

46. Date of Accident (MM/DD/CCYY)

47. Auto Accident State

TREATING DENTIST AND TREATMENT LOCATION INFORMATION

53. I hereby certify that the procedures as indicated by date are in progress (for procedures that require multiple visits) or have been completed.

X _____
Signed (Treating Dentist)   Date

54. NPI

55. License Number

56. Address, City, State, Zip Code

56A. Provider Specialty Code

57. Phone Number ( ) –

58. Additional Provider ID

©2006 American Dental Association
J400 (Same as ADA Dental Claim Form – J401, J402, J403, J404)

To reorder call 1-800-947-4746 or go online at www.adacatalog.org

ADA American Dental Association®
America's leading advocate for oral health

Comprehensive completion instructions for the ADA Dental Claim Form are found in the current version of the CDT manual published by the ADA. Five relevant extracts from that manual follow.

GENERAL INSTRUCTIONS

A. The form is designed so that the name and address (Item 3) of the third-party payer receiving the claim (insurance company/dental benefit plan) is visible in a #10 window envelope. Please fold the form using the 'tick-marks' printed in the margin.

B. In the upper right of the form, a blank space is provided for the convenience of the payer or insurance company, to allow the assignment of a claim or control number.

C. All items in the form must be completed unless it is noted on the form or in the following instructions that completion is not required.

D. When a name and address field is required, the full name of an individual or a full business name, address and zip code must be entered.

E. All dates must include the four-digit year.

F. If the number of procedures reported exceeds the number of lines available on one claim form, the remaining procedures must be listed on a separate, fully completed claim form.

COORDINATION OF BENEFITS (COB)

When a claim is being submitted to the secondary payer, complete the form in its entirety and attach the primary payer's Explanation of Benefits (EOB) showing the amount paid by the primary payer. You may indicate the amount the primary carrier paid in the "Remarks" field (Item # 35).

NATIONAL PROVIDER IDENTIFIER (NPI)

49 and 54   NPI (National Provider Identifier): This is an identifier assigned by the federal government to all providers considered to be HIPAA covered entities. Dentists who are not covered entities may elect to obtain an NPI at their discretion, or may be enumerated if required by a participating provider agreement with a third-party payer or applicable state law/regulation. An NPI is unique to an individual dentist (Type 1 NPI) or dental entity (Type 2 NPI), and has no intrinsic meaning. Additional information on NPI and enumeration can be obtained from the ADA Web site, www.ada.org/goto/npi.

ADDITIONAL PROVIDER IDENTIFIER

52A and 58   Additional Provider ID: This is an identifier assigned to the billing dentist or dental entity other than a Social Security Number (SSN) or Tax Identification Number (TIN). It is not the provider's NPI. The additional identifier is sometimes referred to as a Legacy Identifier (LID). LIDs may not be unique as they are assigned by different entities (e.g., third-party payer; federal government). Some Legacy IDs have an intrinsic meaning.

PROVIDER SPECIALTY CODES

56A   Provider Specialty Code: Enter the code that indicates the type of dental professional who delivered the treatment. Available codes describing treating dentists are listed below. The general code listed as 'Dentist' may be used instead of any other dental practitioner code.

Category / Description Code	Code
Dentist A dentist is a person qualified by a doctorate in dental surgery (D.D.S.) or dental medicine (D.M.D.) licensed by the state to practice dentistry, and practicing within the scope of that license.	122300000X
General Practice	1223G0001X
Dental Specialty (see following list)	Various
Dental Public Health	1223D0001X
Endodontics	1223E0200X
Orthodontics	1223X0400X
Pediatric Dentistry	1223P0221X
Periodontics	1223P0300X
Prosthodontics	1223P0700X
Oral & Maxillofacial Pathology	1223P0106X
Oral & Maxillofacial Radiology	1223D0008X
Oral & Maxillofacial Surgery	1223S0112X

Dental provider taxonomy codes listed above are a subset of the full code set that is posted at: **www.wpc-edi.com/codes/taxonomy**

Should there be any updates to ADA Dental Claim Form completion instructions, the updates will be posted on the ADA's Web site at: **www.ada.org/goto/dentalcode**

Reporting NPI on the ADA Dental Claim Form

ADA Claim Form – Billing Dentist

The ADA paper claim form was updated in 2006 to accommodate reporting NPI. Box 49, which was previously labeled "Provider ID" is now used for the NPI. This box will contain both Type I and Type II NPI numbers depending on status of the billing entity. A new box, 52A, was added to allow the use of an additional identification number. Third party assigned ID numbers previously (legacy ID) may be reported in this box.

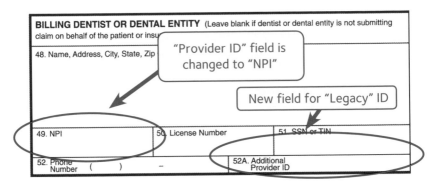

ADA Claim Form – Treating Dentist

Dentists providing treatment may also report their NPI. Box 54, which previously contained the "Provider Specialty Code," is now used for NPI. This box should only contain Type I NPI numbers. The Provider Specialty Code will now be reported in new box 56A. A new box, 58, has also been added to accommodate legacy identifiers and other provider IDs.

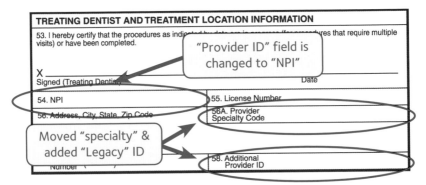

Dental Claim Attachments

Third-party payers sometimes require that supplemental materials accompany claims for payment. These may most commonly include radiographs, periodontal records, narratives, models or primary payer explanations-of-benefits (EOB). Occasionally dentists may wish to submit additional materials to expedite claim adjudication, for example intraoral photographs. Paper claims submitted through the mail may simply have these items "attached." Increasingly, payers are accepting the attachment of images and written materials electronically.

Images:

Dental benefit plans have traditionally requested radiographs for review to validate claims and contain costs. Duplicate radiographs are customarily attached to paper claims and submitted at the request of carrier reviewers. ADA policy emphasizes that dentists should submit duplicate copies of images to third-party payers. Dentists should maintain an original set of radiographs with the chart at all times in order to protect themselves from untoward legal exposure. The ADA also urges third-party payers to only request images when there is a necessity for review by a licensed dentist and return the submitted images in a timely manner. In order to simplify the processing of claims, numerous carriers are reducing or eliminating their requests for radiographs and oral images.

The advent of digital imaging has greatly improved the ease with which oral images are duplicated and transmitted. DICOM (**D**igital **I**maging and **CO**mmunication in **M**edicine) is the standard for communicating medical and dental images and related patient information. The ADA has adopted DICOM as the standard for image communication in dentistry. The DICOM standard allows dental images and other relevant patient data to be communicated not only to third-party payers, but also from one healthcare provider to another. Digitized images may be transmitted electronically through a clearinghouse or directly over the Internet.

Periodontal Claim Attachments:

Adopted in July 2006, the American National Standards Institute (ANSI)/ADA Specification 1047 for Standard Content of a Periodontal Attachment clarifies what clinical information dental offices should send to third-party payers when submitting a periodontal code. Historically, dentists have been required by payers to attach more documentation for periodontal claims than other claims. For that reason, the periodontal attachment standard was the first attachment standard developed by the ADA Standards Committee on Dental Informatics (SCDI). SCDI WG10 is a working group, which includes representatives of practitioner and payer companies and organizations. The ADA develops standards for dental informatics through the SCDI working groups.

Documentation requirements in Specification 1047 are established for each periodontal procedure code found in the ADA's *Code on Dental Procedures and Nomenclature,* as published in the CDT manual. The SCDI standards process allows for revisions to the periodontal procedure codes as published in subsequent editions of the CDT manual. According to the ADA Division of Dental Practice, the standard seeks to:

- facilitate timely claims adjudication for various periodontal procedures;

- take advantage of information technology to increase use of electronic transactions;

- reduce the costs associated with claims processing by providing integrated and interoperable information exchange.

A copy of ANSI/ADA Specification 1047 for Standard Content of a Periodontal Attachment is now available from the ADA through the ADA Product Catalog at www.adacatalog.org.

Narratives:
Attaching a narrative may be done at the request of a third-party payer, but dentists may also wish to include narrative information to satisfy the requirements of a "by report" code or to provide additional information to clarify the details of an out of the ordinary claim. Narratives should include supplementary information that is pertinent to the determination of benefits, or which is required by the third-party payer. Short narratives can be included in the remarks section of the ADA claim form (box 35) or in the Remarks field of an electronic claim.

A narrative should describe the procedure performed and, if applicable, explain the necessity for extra time, use of new technology, etc. Codes that require a report may specify information that should be included in the narrative. When a multi-page narrative is submitted on paper, the patient's name should be included on each page and all pages should be stapled together.

"Top 10" Claim Submission and Processing Concerns

8

CDT
Companion

Chapter 8 – "Top 10" Claim Submission and Processing Concerns

The ADA's Council on Dental Benefit Programs continually receives and addresses a variety of dental claim submission and adjudication questions from member dentists and practice staff. Patterns develop over time and frequently voiced concerns set the stage for discussions between CDBP and third-party payers. This interaction led to a series of *ADA News* articles that examined, from perspectives from ADA members, National Association of Dental Plan members and the Council on Dental Benefit Programs, specific claim submission and adjudication issues such as bundling, delays, lost attachments, overpayment requests, post utilization review, provider contract issues and more.

This series of articles is reprinted in the CDT Companion for ready reference by dentists and their staff. Topics addressed in each article are listed in the table below. Parts 1 through 11 are subjects posed by the ADA; Part 12 is the first of series of subjects posed by NADP.

ADA News often contains articles concerning claim submission and third-party payer issues. These articles are intended to inform dentists of new or changing practices, as well as to provide guidance on how to respond or to obtain additional information.

Text from the published articles are on the pages that follow.

Part	Publication Date	Subject(s)
1.	November 27, 2006	• D4341, D4342 coding for periodontal scaling and root planing (SRP), per quadrant or partial quadrant • D4910 coding for periodontal maintenance
2.	January 8, 2007	• D2950 core buildup, including any pins • Pre-authorizations
3.	March 5, 2007	• Claims processing delays
4.	May 9, 2007	• Claims payment concerns - lost radiographs, claim forms and attachments
5.	June 20, 2007	• Bundling and downcoding
6.	September 20, 2007	• Least expensive alternative treatment clause
7.	February 04, 2008	• Overpayment/refund requests
8.	May 12, 2008	• Coordination of benefits
9.	July 16, 2008	• Provider contract issues – - Carriers' Processing Policies - Billing for Component and Denied Procedures - All Affiliated Carriers - Removal From Network Lists - Specific Provider Service Representative Contracts
10.	September 18, 2008	• Assignment of benefits to participating dentists only
11.	October 20, 2008	• Post-utilization review
12.	December 17, 2009	• Single claim form

Part 1:
November 27, 2006

ADA, NADP share views on dentists' concerns

Dental claims denials were among the most frequent concerns ADA members complained about to the ADA during 2005.

The topic kicks off a series of *ADA News* articles on dentists' "Top 10" concerns submitted to the ADA about their dental claims. These articles will include perspectives from ADA members, National Association of Dental Plan members and the Council on Dental Benefit Programs on specific issues.

"This series of *ADA News* articles grew out of CDBP discussions with NADP about our members' most frequent complaints," said Dr. Alan E. Friedel, chair of the council. "CDBP is working with NADP and the payer industry to facilitate communication to eliminate some of the problems our members and patients are experiencing. We want to clarify what information is necessary to adjudicate claims in a timely manner and consistent fashion."

The Council on Dental Benefit Programs maintains a close watch on industry trends, tracks complaints from members and, when appropriate, works with individual companies to seek solutions.

NADP member companies represent some 82 percent of the estimated 163 million Americans covered by dental benefit plans. Dr. Preddis Sullivan, of NADP's Professional Relations Commission, commented that while no one response can fully reflect the breadth of all plan designs and benefit adjudication requirements, the NADP developed a broad overview on claims denials overall.

"Responding to dentists' concerns required complex information collection, as well as broad circulation of the responses to dental plan members," said Evelyn F. Ireland about the topics to be covered in the series. The NADP executive director said, "We did this to assure the NADP perspective reflects, to the extent possible, the diversity of plans and products of its members and the dental benefits industry overall."

This installment features two topics falling under dental claims denials. An upcoming issue of *ADA News* will feature two more. Subsequent articles will cover the remaining "Top 10" concerns, which include bundling, processing delays, lost attachments, overpayment requests, post utilization review, provider contract issues and more.

D4341, D4342 CODING FOR PERIODONTAL SCALING AND ROOT PLANING (SRP), PER QUADRANT OR PARTIAL QUADRANT

Dental benefits industry perspective

Payers' standard clinical policies relating to coverage of specific procedures are developed based on a review of the scientific literature, the experience of their dental professionals, dental advisory councils and claims histories. A payer's standard practice in an area such as SRP may be modified for a particular employer based on that employer's preferred or negotiated benefit design, analysis of the employer's claims history, or recommendations of their benefits consultant. Thus, two claims to the same payer with a similar patient profile may be treated differently based on the employers' group dental policy under which each patient is covered.

While a pocket depth of 4mm or greater is the most commonly recognized indicator in the literature for SRP, there are differences within dentistry and dental literature about the specifics of pocket depths as benchmarks. Thus, payers establish their own criteria based on all these factors which can differ from payer to payer and potentially, from one customer to another within a single payer's book of business.

Just as payers' clinical policies differ, claims for periodontal procedures and treatments are frequently subject to coding variations when submitted by dentists. The addition of code D4342 has been helpful in determining appropriate benefit reimbursements. In the past, when code D4341 (full quadrant) was the only SRP code, it was more difficult to determine coverage where diagnostics supported SRP for a small number of teeth in a quadrant.

The use of D4341 or D4342 in reporting more than 2 quadrants within a single dental visit will usually trigger a request for additional information such as a full-mouth periodontal charting, full-mouth X-ray, periodontal diagnosis and the treatment plan.

Many payers now post their guidelines to their Web sites (usually in a member protected area due to the inclusion of CDT codes which are copyright protected), include them in the provider office reference guide or make them available to dentists on request.

Tips for minimizing claim denials or delays for SRP:

- Before submitting a claim for SRP, check the company's guidelines on their Web site or in the provider office reference guide.
- When submitting SRP for more than 2 quadrants within a single visit, include documentation—full-mouth periodontal charting, FMX, periodontal diagnosis and the treatment plan. ∎

D4341, D4342 CODING FOR PERIODONTAL SCALING AND ROOT PLANING (SRP), PER QUADRANT OR PARTIAL QUADRANT

Dentist perspective

Many dentists don't understand why claims for SRP are denied when the patient has abnormal pocket depths. A claim may be paid on a patient with 4mm pockets while at other times the same payer may deny the same procedure for another patient who had the same or similar clinical presentation.

This is very confusing for dentists. When the claim is denied some patients may think that the dentist is performing unnecessary procedures.

When patients or members of the dental office staff contact a payer to determine whether a benefit is available under a specific plan, they are usually given a yes/no response. Specific payment guidelines may not be provided. If these were provided, the process would be much more transparent and many of these situations could be avoided. Until this is common practice, the carrier should make it clear to both patients and dentists that while SRP may be necessary, their plan will only provide a benefit when the plan's particular clinical indicators are present. If third-party payers disclosed the actual payment parameters, dentists could then tell the patient in advance what the plan might cover.

The ADA Council on Dental Benefit Programs notes that a single payer can reimburse various employee groups differently. In some cases payers act as insurers. In other cases they simply administer a policy on behalf of an employer. Purchasers of plans that cover many lives can often negotiate changes in reimbursement rates to meet economic targets. Dentists should advise their patients that coverage is often based on employer funding of the policy purchased rather than the clinical need of the specific patient. ■

Dental benefits industry perspective

Quite frankly, this code is a challenge for benefits administrators as well. In order to appropriately determine the benefit for procedure code D4910, it is necessary to have knowledge of the patients' prior periodontal history. Often, this information is not available during claims processing. If the patient has no prior claim history with the payer, or previous periodontal services were not paid by the current payer, it is difficult to properly assess the benefits level available to the patient.

If you are aware that the current payer does not have previous periodontal history on a patient, submitting periodontal charting with the claim will assist in the determination of benefits. Since most payers electronically store claim forms, submitted diagnostics and electronic attachments, an existing record will reside with the payer should there be any question as to the handling of the benefits reimbursement. Thus, resubmission of diagnostic materials would not be necessary on a patient whose periodontal therapy was covered by the payer.

Many payers require an examination, targeted periodontal probing, and a periodontal diagnosis for reimbursement of code D4910. As stated in the *Code on Dental Procedures and Nomenclature*, this procedure is instituted after periodontal therapy.

Although no time frame is outlined in the CDT, most payers require a waiting period of 8 to 12 weeks. If there are unusual circumstances that would require a different interval of treatment, documentation by the dentist with the original claim submission should forestall requests for additional information to determine the patient's benefits.

At times, payers are limited by specific guidelines from employer group and dental group contract language. When plan limitations exist, and continued D4910 are reported, many payers will allow payment for an adult prophylaxis, which is an integral component of the more global D4910, to provide some level of coverage for the insured patient.

Tips for minimizing claim denials for periodontal maintenance:

- If there are unusual circumstances that require a different interval of treatment than the one specified in the patient's plan documents, the dentist should provide documentation with the original claim submission.
- If a patient is covered under a new group policy, submission of the patient's history of treatment with the initial claim for D4910 will assist in the determination. ∎

Dentist perspective

According to the Code on Dental Procedures and Nomenclature, this procedure is performed following periodontal therapy and continues for the life of the dentition. Periodontal maintenance is often denied, however, because many carriers have limited benefits for this procedure. Reports received from our member dentists indicate that some payers have limited this procedure to being paid as a benefit only within 2 to 12 months of SRP.

No mention of a time period following periodontal treatment is provided in the Code. Some payers have qualified periodontal maintenance by denying benefits for this procedure unless two or more quadrants have received prior therapy.

It seems that each carrier has different policies/limitations for this procedure. This is very confusing for both dentists and patients. While the dentist is performing and reporting the correct procedure, benefits are denied solely because of the plan's limitations. However, absent a full explanation that accompanies the denial, the patient may think that the dentist is incorrectly reporting or performing dental procedures. Disclosure of the processing policies in the employee benefit booklet and in an Explanation of Benefits would be very helpful to avoid inadvertent negative implications with respect to the doctor-patient treatment. Allowance of an alternate benefit for a lesser procedure should also be disclosed in the benefit booklet and the EOB.

The ADA Council on Dental Benefits believes it is incumbent upon dentists to deliver appropriate care to patients based upon clinical need, not by third party reimbursement that may be forthcoming. After periodontal therapy has been completed, newly exposed root structure and altered architecture often make debridement of plaque and calculus more difficult. This does not change with time.

Patients should be told in advance that plan provisions may not provide for reimbursement of D4910 for extended periods. We must code for what we do, and educate our patients that all procedures are not covered by all plans. ■

Part 2
January 08, 2007

ADA, NADP share views on dentists' concerns

This is the second installment of a series of *ADA News* articles on dentists' "Top 10" concerns submitted to the ADA about their dental claims. These articles include perspectives from ADA members, National Association of Dental Plan members and the Council on Dental Benefit Programs.

Dental claims denials were among the most frequent concerns ADA members complained about to the ADA during 2005.

Two more topics under dental claims denials were featured in the Nov. 20, 2006 *ADA News*. Subsequent articles will cover the remaining nine of the "Top 10" concerns, which include claims processing delays, lost attachments, provider contract issues and others.

D2950 CORE BUILDUP, INCLUDING ANY PINS

Dental benefits industry perspective

Both this code and D6973 core buildup for retainer, including any pins, creates problems for payers. Some of the problems result from limitations in an employer's group policy and some result from lack of documentation to support use of this procedure in addition to a crown.

The change in the descriptor in CDT-4 clarified the procedure, however all claims submissions are not consistent with the descriptor. In the description it states the procedure, "Refers to building up of anatomical crown when restorative crown will be placed, whether or not pins are used. A material is placed in the tooth preparation for a crown when there is insufficient tooth strength and retention for the crown procedure. This should not be reported when the procedure only involves a filler to eliminate any undercut, box form or concave irregularity in the preparation."

Some payers find that buildups are reported in addition to a crown procedure when there is a base placed only to restore undercuts and tooth structure that is removed during the crown preparation. This is contrary to the descriptor for this code. Under this definition, a dental consultant acting on behalf of the payer may decide, based on the documentation submitted, that the reported crown buildup did not meet the definition and is a part of the crown procedure. Thus, only the crown procedure will be reimbursed.

(Continued on p.138)

D2950 CORE BUILDUP, INCLUDING ANY PINS

Dentist perspective

Many complaints concerning the denial of core buildups were brought to the attention of the ADA Council on Dental Benefit Programs. Dentists perform this procedure when it is necessary prior to restoring a tooth with a crown. Complaints centered on the lack of a benefit for this procedure. Some dentists complained that this procedure is bundled with a crown procedure.

Bundling of separate procedures to limit a benefit is against ADA policy. If a plan chooses to bundle these procedures, the plan should allow the sum of the fees for the crown and the crown buildup as the total fee for the procedure and provide the appropriate benefit. Dentists do not always understand the parameters for payment by plan. Patients should be clearly informed as to benefit limitations and it should be made clear in the benefit booklet and explanation of benefits that plan limitations and not clinical necessity determine payments.

CDBP notes that many patients do not understand how their dental benefits really function. They do not understand that dentists who attempt to deliver ideal care may find that the constraints of a given policy do not align with the treatment plan. It is incumbent on us to give appropriate care notwithstanding a patient's insurance coverage. This is an example of just such a situation. We cannot interpret the meaning of any code beyond what it actually states.

The payers who choose not to fund for core buildups do so for many reasons. Having patients who understand the limitations of their plan prior to treatment can avoid problems.

Regarding explanation of benefit language, CDBP works very hard to help insurance companies find language which is not only succinct but which does not infer bad faith on the part of the dentist. We have had some success in this regard by direct correspondence with individual companies.

It is incumbent upon the dentist to help the patient understand the clinical basis for treatment, in spite of contractual limitations by the plan. In doing so, the rationale for the core buildup to improve retention form and improve the clinical outcome is clearly explained for the benefit of the patient. In cases of denial, it may be appropriate to submit an appeal outlining the reasons for the procedure, leading to improved prognosis. ■

Dental benefits industry perspective *(Continued from p.136)*

Benefit limitations are required, under state law or in the case of Taft-Hartley contracts under negotiated labor agreements, to be disclosed in plan documents that are provided to insured patients. These documents must meet readability standards which are most often at the grade school reading level and sometimes are required in foreign languages as well. While these plan documents are made available to insured patients, they may be lost or misplaced and thus not referenced by the patient when seeking treatment.

EOB* language is intended to be succinct yet descriptive of the payers' action relating to the patient's claim. Payers are often limited in the space provided for explanations and use shortened descriptions to convey information. When such language results in misunderstandings between the patient and the dentist, payers are open to suggestions for changes in language.

Tip to minimize claim denials for core buildup:

In the initial claim submission, documentation of the condition that resulted in the buildup should be provided, if applicable.

*The National Association of Dental Plans has recently distributed to its members the ADA Council on Dental Benefit Programs' summary, "ADA Position on Content of Explanation of Benefits (EOB) Statements." ■

D2950 CORE BUILDUP, INCLUDING ANY PINS

Dentist perspective

(See page 137)

Dental benefits industry perspective

The complexity of dental benefits is market driven. However, employee benefits booklets and disclosure statements are required by state laws to be written at a grade school reading level and in some instances provided in languages other than English to facilitate patient understanding.

The involvement of the dentist in explaining benefits to patients varies by dental product.

In dental health maintenance organizations, network dentists are provided with a manual or Web site access that lists covered benefits and patient payment obligations. Since there is no routine claims process for DHMOs, there is an expectation that the dental office is explaining charges for covered services (co-payments) and non-covered services when they are completing treatment.

For dental preferred provider organizations (roughly half of the market today) and dental indemnity plans (about 26 percent of the market), payers do not expect dentists or their office staff to explain covered benefits to the patient. While dentists may elect to provide general information about benefits based on their experience, payers make specific information available to patients through their Web sites, benefit booklets and customer service lines.

"Preauthorization" and "predetermination" are processes that payers make available to dentists to clearly determine the potential benefits for a specific patient. These are distinct and different terms and processes which are outlined in many state statutes. They are not interchangeable. ("Pre-approved" is not a term generally used by payers.)

Many DHMO plans require preauthorization prior to referral to a specialist so that the plan can review the treatment prescribed and authorize payment. However, even with a DHMO, eligibility must still be established at time of service for a benefit to be covered.

Most DPPO and dental indemnity plans do not require preauthorization but offer a voluntary predetermination of benefits process. This is a service to the dentist or patient to determine prior to treatment what their plan will cover and reimburse for the course of treatment presented if the patient does two things:

1. remains eligible;

2. has not exhausted the plan maximum at the time of service.

(Continued on p.142)

Dentist perspective

Although it is incumbent upon patients to understand their coverage, many times the policies are not easily understood by lay people. It can be time consuming for the dental office to first learn about and then explain the terms of any particular policy to a patient. Also, since policies can change at the beginning of a plan year, this can make it very difficult for any dentist to understand how they will be paid for any procedure. Dentists use the pre-authorization process to determine a patient's coverage.

Sometimes a treatment plan has been pre-authorized or pre-approved by the carrier and the treatment is performed by the dentist with the expectation that the claim will be paid, but it is denied. The reasons for denial vary, such as the patient is no longer eligible, the maximum allowable has been paid or time limitations have been exceeded. The pre-authorization should clearly indicate that the pre-authorization is not a guarantee of payment.

The ADA Council on Dental Benefit Programs believes that if at all possible, patients should be empowered to get paper or internet copies of benefit booklets and policy guidelines so they can make informed decisions.

When a preauthorization is received in one calendar year and is begun in the next, there is always the potential for a problem.

The slow turnaround on a preauthorization often creates frustration for patient and practitioner. The process can be used to uncover proposed treatment which is not covered or is disallowed. Patients must understand the benefit outlined in the preauthorization is tempered by the allowable benefits at the time of service, not the time of preauthorization submission. ■

Dental benefits industry perspective *(Continued from p.141)*

Most carriers do clearly note on these forms of advice about potential coverage that the estimated payments for services are not guaranteed. Whether it is a preauthorization or a predetermination (sometimes called pre-estimate), it is based on the eligibility and remaining benefits at the time it was issued. If a member loses coverage or other benefits are paid in the time between the preauthorization or predetermination and the submission of a claim, benefits would change.

Dental insurance is like other types of insurance, the actual coverage is determined on the date of occurrence. If any eligibility of coverage has changed, the benefits are adjusted accordingly.

Tips to minimize claim denials and promote patient understanding of benefits:

- Encourage patients to contact their payer directly through customer service lines to verify benefits for particular procedures.

- Submit predeterminations on complex, costly procedures as close to the date of proposed service as possible. ■

Part 3
March 05, 2007

ADA, NADP share views on claims processing delays

'Steps should be taken to ensure that payments are as prompt as possible'

This is the third installment of a series of ADA News articles on dentists' "Top 10" concerns submitted to the ADA about their dental claims. These articles include perspectives from ADA members, National Association of Dental Plan members and the Council on Dental Benefit Programs.

Claims processing delays and requests by payers for additional information were among the most frequent concerns ADA members complained about to the ADA during 2005.

Dentist and dental benefits industry perspectives on dental claims denials were featured in the Nov. 20, 2006, and Jan. 8 ADA News.

Subsequent articles will cover the remaining nine of the "Top 10" concerns, which include lost attachments, bundling and down-coding, post utilization review, assignments to participating doctors only, provider contract issues and others.

Dental benefits industry perspective

Payers are aware of the importance of claims payments to dentists. The dental insurance industry processes more than 250 million claims annually with about 70 percent being auto-adjudicated, which means processed with computerized decision logic that is linked to the provisions of an employers' group policy. Auto-adjudication is used with both electronic claims and paper claims to improve processing speed and identify claims that require staff review. Paper claims are either scanned or keyed into the system. Handwritten entries on claim forms, light print or unclear copies may result in some information not being captured from the original paper submission. As in any system, the complexities involved in claims processing can create misunderstandings as well as break down.

Regulations and employer group requirements: Payers are regulated by the states for prompt payment of claims. This is not only required by law in many states, but is actually part of performance guarantees mandated by many large employer groups.

Performance guarantees are a tool by which these employers identify claim processing timeliness and accuracy rates which the payer must meet. Failure to do so results in penalties, such as financial fines or loss of the employer as a client.

In self-funded situations, employers determine covered benefits and how quickly claims are processed and paid since the employer's money is at risk. About 37 million Americans are enrolled in dental plans through employer self-funded groups. This is 26 percent of the private market for dental benefits. In these cases, the payer performs as a dental administrator and is obligated by contract to process claims within the time frame specified. These groups are regulated under federal law—Employee Retirement Income Security Act of 1974—not state law.

Industry data shows that 93 percent of all dental claims are processed within 10 days—well below the time required under the typical state "clean claim" laws. Payers do not want to handle claims multiple times nor is there an advantage in delaying payment because delays:

- add to the cost of administration;
- create complaints from dental offices and consumers;
- impede the payer's ability to meet performance guarantees.

Claims processing pitfalls: The ADA claim form is the prime document that conveys what was done, when and to whom, and acts as the bill to ensure the

(Continued on p.146)

Dentist perspective

Insurance payments are a key component in the income stream for many dentists, and when prompt payment is not received, dentists may have trouble paying staff and other administrative expenses.

The Council on Dental Benefit Programs believes that once professional care has been delivered to the patient the dentist deserves prompt financial compensation. Delayed or denied insurance payments may already affect the dentist-patient relationship; steps should be taken to ensure that payments are as prompt as possible.

Although 46 states have prompt-pay laws, those laws apply only to "clean claims," or claims submitted to third-party payers without any missing or wrong information. Many times clean claims are rejected for missing claim information that is clearly written on the claim form. Many dentists consider this a stall tactic by the insurance company in order to delay the payment to them.

Third-party payers often dispute claims on the basis that services were not necessary or that a different procedure should have been done. Payment is delayed until the dentist provides additional information. Often the carrier asks for more information or clarification of the information submitted. Resubmitting these claims is often a time-consuming and costly process for the dental office.

According to CDBP, any delay in claims payment is compounded by the cost of collection activities, bad debt ratio, as well as the time value of money to the practice.

The ADA, through the CDBP, has been working with the NADP to try to improve the efficiency and speed of claims settlements and thus improve dentist-patient, patient-carrier and dentist-carrier relationships. The ultimate goal has been to reduce unnecessary and unsolicited submissions, which is a growing problem and expense for dentists and carriers.

Many dentists believe that all claims should be thoroughly reviewed before a request for additional information is sent to the dentist. They also believe that when a consultant requests additional information to process the claim, the claim processing should be expedited once that information is received. ■

Dental benefits industry perspective *(Continued from p.144)*

dentist is paid. The clear and complete form should result in prompt and accurate reimbursement. Payers find that some common information which is needed for the adjudication process and coordination of benefits is often missing.

It is also common for periodontal charting and X-rays to be missing from claims (when required). Payers recognize that it can be difficult to check each payer's requirements for attachments. NADP has partnered with National Electronic Attachment, Inc. to create a single online portal for dental offices to check payer attachment requirements. This portal, NEA FastLook, was launched in January and can be found at www.nea-fast.com.

In addition to missing attachments it is not unusual for a payer to receive claims with outdated Code on Dental Procedures and Nomenclature codes. This requires that the claim be reconciled to CDT 2007 which payers are required to use under federal HIPAA law and can cause delays.

Another common claim submission error is for the payer name or code to be reported incorrectly. This may be due to outdated practice management software or submitting through vendors that have not updated their lists. One clearinghouse reported that 9,258 claims were submitted by 3,883 dental offices in one month under a payer name or code that had not existed for more than five years. Clearinghouses have created databases to get these claims into the system, but the use of out-dated information does create delays for some claims.

Another issue payers face is receiving claims for other payers. Often this results from mailing large batches of claims in a single envelope. To comply with privacy laws, the payer must return these claims directly to the dentist.

Reviews for dental necessity: In limited instances (less than 5 percent of claims) there may need to be a review for dental necessity. Dental necessity is a provision in many dental benefit policies, but may not be utilized by every payer. Some payers have dental directors or dental consultants who are licensed dentists to review specific claims. A discussion of claims denials was published in the Nov. 20, 2006 ADA News. The most common reasons for denying a claim for dental necessity are extraction of asymptomatic third molars, osseous surgery in the absence of sufficient pocketing/bone loss, and crown buildup when enough tooth structure is present to retain the crown.

(Continued on p.148)

Dentist perspective

(See page 145)

Dental benefits industry perspective *(Continued from p.146)*

Requests for additional information such as X-rays, further narratives and diagnostic materials usually occur when there is some question on a particular procedure or this information is not initially submitted. When this need arises it is not because payers are trying to discern the course of treatment, but do need to know if the procedure performed falls within the definition of the patient's coverage.

Similarly reviews for dental necessity are not intended to interfere or disagree with the clinical judgment of the attending dentist but rather to identify whether the procedure performed falls within the parameters of the patient's coverage. ∎

ADA/NADP share views on claims payment concerns

This is the fourth installment of a series of *ADA News* articles on dentists' "Top 10" concerns submitted to the ADA about their dental claims. These articles include perspectives from ADA members, National Association of Dental Plans members and the Council on Dental Benefit Programs.

Lost radiographs, claim forms and attachments were among the most frequent concerns ADA members complained about to the ADA during 2005.

Dentist and dental benefits industry perspectives on claims processing delays were covered in the March 5 *ADA News*. Dental claims denials were featured in the Nov. 20, 2006, and Jan. 8 *ADA News*.

Subsequent articles will feature the remaining "Top 10" concerns which include bundling and down-coding, post utilization review, assignments to participating doctors only, provider contract issues and others.

LOST RADIOGRAPHS, CLAIM FORMS AND ATTACHMENTS

Dental benefits industry perspective

Some X-rays and claims may be lost from the sheer volume of handling 250 million claims annually. About 70 percent of all claims are submitted on paper. Paper processes require manual systems that can fail. Mistakes are inherent in all systems.

Carriers have introduced a variety of systems to reduce the paperwork of claims and minimize mistakes such as lost attachments.

These include:

- scanning all paper and X-rays into electronic systems;
- reducing or eliminating the need for submission of X-rays;
- establishing auto-adjudication systems;
- promoting the use of electronic transactions.

Additionally, in response to discussions of the ADA/NADP Joint Working Group on Radiograph return, NADP recognized the difficulty for a dental office keeping track of varied carrier attachment requirements. NADP worked with a commercial vendor, National Electronic Attachment, to create a single Web-based portal where carrier attachment requirements can be accessed. The portal, called FastLook, was launched in January 2007 at "www.neafast.com". For information on NEA services call 1-800-782-5150.

In some instances, the method by which claims are submitted increases the possibility of loss. Attachments that are not firmly affixed to a claim form can get separated when the mail is opened; this is especially true when multiple claims are submitted in one envelope. If X-rays are not labeled and get detached from claims, they cannot always be matched back to the appropriate claim form. Privacy and security standards require that personal medical information be protected, so unmatched attachments would most likely be destroyed.

When a payer does not require an X-ray for a claim, the process established by that payer may require that the X-ray be removed and returned or destroyed. If a subsequent issue removes the claim from auto-adjudication for review, an X-ray may be requested at that time.

Submitting electronic claims and the appropriate attachments to them is the best way to avoid the loss of claims, X-rays and other attachments. Many of those offices that do submit claims electronically do not have the equipment necessary to submit X-rays as electronic attachments. Given this circumstance and the fact that some 60 to 70 percent of dental claims are still submitted as paper correspondence, it is important that payers and dentists develop processes to minimize the potential of lost claim forms and attachments. ∎

LOST RADIOGRAPHS, CLAIM FORMS AND ATTACHMENTS

Dentist perspective

One of the biggest complaints concerning third-party claim payment is lost claims and lost X-rays. Many dentists report sending in claims or X-rays several times before the insurance company will acknowledge receipt. Often X-rays are submitted with the claim, but the dentist will receive an explanation of benefits requesting the X-rays.

Confusion often arises due to the lack of standardization for attachments from carriers and the inability to reference attachment requirements for multiple carriers in a central location. This mandates that each office contact each carrier individually to determine what is needed to adjudicate the claim. In the absence of definitive information, the dental office often submits additional attachments to avoid possible delays in payment by a subsequent additional request.

The Council on Dental Benefit Programs notes that there is no uniformity within the payer community regarding submission of radiographs, partly due to different business structures within the industry. Some companies would prefer that no radiographs be sent unless they are requested. Others want to see images at the time specific procedure codes are reported.

The council says that the underlying concern from the industry perspective is based upon a cost versus benefit relationship. Is the additional cost for having the radiographs sent with a claim and then returned offset by a savings gained by reducing potentially fraudulent claims? Each company makes these and other similar decisions on its own. This proprietary information can help determine the profitability of any given payer. When bidding for contracts it provides some companies with a competitive advantage. For this reason, payers do not share this information, and this is why standardizing of third parties' handling of claims is such a daunting task. The more things become standardized, the more each company looks alike, and the harder it becomes to distinguish them in the marketplace.

If X-rays are submitted together with a paper claim, how do they get separated? What happens to all those lost X-rays? In addition, many electronic claims submissions require attachments to be mailed separately because of dental offices' inability to scan paper forms and standard radiographs through the practice management software. This delays claim processing and increases the risk for error.

Many dentists think that losing claims and X-rays are delay tactics used by third-party payers in order for them to meet financial or claim processing goals. Although claims processing delays have a cost to payers as well, some dentists believe that the financial benefit to payers outweighs those costs. ■

Part 5
June 20, 2007

ADA/NADP share views on bundling and downcoding

This is the fifth installment of a series of *ADA News* articles on dentists' "Top 10" concerns submitted to the ADA about dental claims. These articles include perspectives from ADA members, National Association of Dental Plans members and the Council on Dental Benefit Programs.

Bundling and downcoding are among the most frequent concerns ADA members complained about to the ADA during 2005. Lost radiographs, claim forms and attachments were covered in the May 7 *ADA News*. Claims processing delays was covered in the March 5 *ADA News*. Dental claims denials were featured in the Nov. 20, 2006, and Jan. 8 *ADA News*.

Subsequent articles will feature the remaining "Top 10" concerns which include post utilization review, assignments to participating doctors only, provider contract issues

---

BUNDLING AND DOWNCODING

Dental benefits industry perspective

Payers agree that both they and dentists have the responsibility to utilize the Code on Dental Procedures and Nomenclature as the designated standard for the reporting of dental services. Through the review and revision process, the Code has evolved to clearly define the scope of dental procedures, at times clarifying component services that may be considered part of another procedure code. One of the most common problems that payers have with claims is the use of outdated versions of CDT. Under the Health Insurance Portability and Accountability Act, payers must utilize the most current version of CDT and claims submitted with outdated procedure codes will be updated to the current codes in CDT.

Bundling:
What is often described as bundling is the effort of payers to follow guidelines established in the Code. For example, payers commonly see claims submitted with the following combinations of services that are not consistent with the Code:

- Pins reported as a separate service from a core buildup (the D2950 buildup code includes pins);

- Adhesives, bases or liners as a separate service from the restorations (the Code defines these to be included as part of the restoration); *(Continued on p.154)*

Dentist perspective

Bundling is defined by the ADA as "The systematic combining of distinct dental procedures by third-party payers that results in a reduced benefit for the patient/beneficiary."

Many dentists want to know what the purpose of developing a procedure coding system with separate codes for distinct dental procedures is when third-party payers simply ignore it. Although there are some instances of bundling due to improper filing of the claim, the instances of concern to dentists are when procedures which are legitimately separate are bundled either inappropriately, or due to contract provisions without explanation.

One of the most common complaints the ADA receives concerning bundling issues pertains to radiographs. Several radiographs will be combined and recoded as a full mouth series and are then subjected to dental benefit plan frequency limitations. Usually the number or type of radiographs taken would not constitute a full mouth series.

Another area of confusion is the practice of some third party payers to combine a panoramic radiograph together with bitewings for payment as a full mouth radiographic examination (FMX). While a panoramic radiograph has many diagnostic uses, its inherent distortion does not permit the clinical differentiation required for many dental procedures.

Downcoding is defined by the ADA as "A practice of third-party payers in which the benefit code has been changed to a less complex and/or lower cost procedure than was reported except where delineated in contract agreements."

When a third-party payer downcodes a procedure, it may be understood by the patient that the payer is making a determination that a lower level of care was needed or should have been provided. Dentists feel that the determination of the level of care necessary for the treatment of their patients should be made by them, not the insurance company. Unless the purely business reason for the payer decision is explained, this may wrongfully interfere with the doctor-patient relationship.

Many carriers typically do not disclose their bundling or downcoding policies, even during the contract negotiation process. Dentists and patients have no way of knowing what the reimbursement will be until the explanation of benefits is received. When the dentist has a contractual arrangement with the carrier, and procedures are bundled or downcoded, a greater dollar amount than what was anticipated may have to be written off. If the dentist is not contracted with the carrier, the patient's coinsurance may also be greater than what they had expected. *(Continued on p.155)*

Dental benefits industry perspective *(Continued from p.152)*

- Occlusal adjustments and minor adjustments to prostheses as a separate service, when the prosthetic service includes routine post-delivery care;

- Suture removal, as a separate service from the extractions, which include suturing and postoperative care; and

- X-rays taken during the course of root canal therapy as a separate service from the root canal, which by definition, includes intra-operative X-rays.

For the examples above, payers will often consider these component services as part of the main procedure in accordance with the Code and pay benefits accordingly.

Regarding X-rays, payers can understand dentists' confusion regarding the coding for a complete radiographic series. The D0210 code for an intraoral complete series (including bitewings) does not specify the number of intraoral films that would compose a full mouth set of radiographs. The FDA provides some guidance by defining a full mouth radiographic examination (FMX) as "a set of intraoral radiographs usually consisting of 14 to 22 periapical and posterior bitewing images intended to display the crowns and roots of all teeth, periapical areas and alveolar bone crest." However, because radiographs are individualized, it is understood that the number of films to adequately view what is defined in a complete series will vary from patient to patient. Thus, payers may establish benefit guidelines that multiple intraoral films on the same date of service will be considered a complete series of intraoral radiographs or will be limited to the maximum reimbursement of an FMX. These guidelines should be available to both dentists and patients.

It is a fairly common occurrence for insurers to receive a panoramic film and bitewings from pediatric dentists and general dentists as their full mouth series. Payers recognize that panorex films alone are not considered sufficient for the diagnosis of decay, and must be accompanied by a set of bitewing X-rays if they are to be used as an aid for full diagnostic purposes. The combination of a set of bitewings and a panoramic film is particularly useful for those patients who are to be referred for orthodontic consult and for extraction of wisdom teeth. The practice of combining these and providing a benefit equal to the full mouth series is a result of requests from the dental community, and not the creation of payers. When a single panoramic film is taken and submitted for orthodontic records, third molar evaluation and similar cases, they are often benefited separately from a full mouth series depending on the employer group. *(Continued on p.156)*

Dentist perspective *(Continued from p.153)*

There is no disagreement about the right of a plan purchaser and the payer to decide what will be covered and what will not be covered. In some cases limits on coverage are an industry response to what payers believe is abuse of the system by some dentists. The concern often goes back to explanation of benefits language. If payers would clearly explain that these are economic decisions between the plan purchaser and the payer in a manner that does not impact the doctor-patient relationship, it would help clear the air. Patients still might not be happy with how the benefits are administered but the dentist would not be held to blame. In the present climate, it is incumbent upon dentists and their staff to explain to patients in advance of treatment that a treatment plan should be dictated by what the doctor and patient determine is clinically appropriate, not by plan compensation.

In addition, carrier coding methodologies should be made readily available to both patients and providers. ■

Dental benefits industry perspective *(Continued from p.154)*

Downcoding:

Most often employers contract for group dental benefits and contribute to the premiums which pay for the dental services provided to their employees. Payers have a responsibility to the employer-purchasers and their employees to assure that appropriate procedure codes are applied to the reported dental services and to make payments under the terms of the contract for those procedure codes. Payers' downcode or recode submitted procedure code(s) to a less complex or lower cost procedure(s) to apply the appropriate procedure codes for dental services based upon professional review of the information submitted by dentists and current CDT descriptors and nomenclature.

An example is a claim received with the reporting of three sites of D4263 (bone replacement graft–first site in quadrant) within the same quadrant. In this situation, payers will recode the two additional D4263 codes to D4264 (bone replacement graft– each additional site in quadrant) in accordance with the Code. Another example is the submission of code D4341 when only one to three teeth are treated in a quadrant. A payer may change the code to D4342 to accurately reflect the procedure being performed.

Payers may also pay benefits for procedures as a result of applying an allowance for benefits in the cases where dental benefit plans have a least expensive alternative treatment provision. In such cases, what may appear as downcoding is a reflection of the insured's specific allowance under their dental benefit plan for benefit determination only. This application of a dental benefit policy provision is not intended to dictate the level of care reported by the dentist, only to provide some benefit to the patient under the policy. The application of a LEAT provision should be clearly noted in the explanation of benefits. Some dental benefit plans allow the dentist to additionally bill the patient for services to which an "alternate benefit or LEAT" provision is applied—those services that the patient and dentist chose as the best option for treatment.

It is important to note that some employer groups may elect to have claims paid exactly as submitted by dentists, but there is obviously a cost to the employer for doing so. Others may set their own guidelines for administration which the payer must follow for that employer group. Again, payers are responsible to administer the benefit allowance for the reporting of dental services in accordance with the contract established with the employer. *(Continued on p.158)*

Dentist perspective

(See page 155)

Dental benefits industry perspective *(Continued from p.156)*

Coverage determination guidelines:

Most payers establish utilization review programs that address both coverage determination guidelines and covered procedures. Appropriately trained staff or licensed professionals are responsible for code adjustment decisions in accordance with these program descriptions as well as compliance with state regulations. Payers vary with respect to their communication of such guidelines to dentists, but most make them available through some means for their insured plans. Since payers often administer plans for self-funded employers that may determine their own reimbursement guidelines, the payer's guidelines may not apply to some employer groups.

Tips:

- Verify procedure codes are appropriately reported in accordance with the current CDT descriptors and nomenclature.
- Contact payers directly for clarification of concerns related to coding of dental services.
- Explain to the patient in advance of treatment by use of pretreatment estimates that a treatment plan should be decided by what the doctor and patient determine is clinically appropriate, not by plan compensation. ■

Part 6
September 20, 2007

ADA/NADP share views on the least expensive alternative treatment clause

This is the sixth installment of a series of *ADA News* articles on dentists' "Top Ten" concerns submitted to the ADA about dental claims. These articles include perspectives from ADA members, National Association of Dental Plans members and the Council on Dental Benefit Programs.

Past *ADA News* issues included articles on claims processing delays, dental claims denials, claim forms and attachments and bundling and downcoding.

Subsequent articles will feature the remaining "Top Ten" concerns, which include post utilization review, assignments to participating doctors and others.

Dental benefits industry perspective

When alternate benefit or LEAT provisions are applied, they are not meant to dictate treatment, question professional judgment or interfere with doctor-patient relationships. The ultimate decision on treatment is up to the dentist and patient. The LEAT provision actually funds a range of treatment options within the reimbursement boundaries established by the employer group contract.

The Surgeon General's Report "Oral Health 2000" found that the top barrier to seeking dental care was cost and that dental benefits overcame that barrier. Dental benefits increase the percentage of people visiting a dentist on an annual basis by at least 20 percent. ("Oral Health 2000" indicates that 70.4 percent of individuals with private dental insurance reported seeing a dentist in the past year, compared to 50.8 percent of those without dental insurance.)

While consumers may not anticipate using their medical benefits, they know they will use their dental benefits annually.

Alternate benefit or LEAT provisions are one component in maintaining dental coverage affordability. A core principal of insurance is the "law of large numbers," which means that there are predictable events with calculable costs over a large population. Identifying potential therapies for the incidences of disease and predicting costs is critical to maintaining the affordability of insurance benefits. Keeping benefits affordable expands access to dental care.

Most dental benefits are provided by employers through group coverage. More of the group dental benefits market is becoming voluntary. (Voluntary means the employer arranged for the group coverage but the employee pays the majority and often 100 percent of the premium.) Overall, most employers are decreasing contributions to employees' dental coverage.

Since dental benefits play an important role in enabling consumers to access dental care but consumers are paying more of the premium cost out-of-pocket, in addition to deductibles and co-payments, it is important to keep the cost of coverage affordable.

An alternate benefit provision in a dental plan contract allows the third-party payer or insurance carrier to determine the benefit based on an alternative procedure that is generally less expensive than the one provided or proposed by the servicing provider. This provision is used as a payment mechanism in dental indemnity and dental preferred provider organization plans to allow claim payment systems to

(Continued on p.162)

Dentist perspective

A type of cost containment measure used by many third-party payers is the least expensive alternative treatment, also known as the least expensive professionally acceptable treatment clause. Under a LEAT clause, when there are multiple viable options of treatment available for a specific condition, the plan will only pay for the least expensive treatment alternative.

Implementation of this cost-containment measure requires that the diagnosis, evaluation and recommendation of the treating dentist be evaluated by the insurance company. ADA policy states "to best educate the public as to the application of this clause when it is applied to limit benefit coverage, the plan should inform the plan purchaser of that application and should provide the patient and treating dentist with the name and qualifications of the individual making the determination, along with the basis for determination that another treatment is in the best interests of the patient and appropriate for the patient's condition." While insurance companies use LEAT review to make benefit funding decisions under a given plan, many dentists find their application potentially confusing to their patients. Some patients may ask if their dentist's professional judgment is being questioned by the insurance company, which then requires additional explanations by the dentist to clear up any confusion.

The most frequently cited examples of LEAT clauses being administered are when composite fillings are alternate benefited to amalgams and when crowns are alternate benefited to large fillings. Although there may be alternative treatments that are clinically acceptable, often the least expensive treatment may not be what is in the best interest of the patient. The most appropriate treatment decision is made directly between the treating doctor and patient, and that decision may be influenced by the insurance company's benefit funding policies based solely on cost savings. It may be true that providing a benefit for a less expensive treatment is better than providing no benefit at all, but it can also be argued that the best benefit to the patient is in funding the procedure that the treating dentist and patient determined is appropriate, based on the clinical circumstances, needs and desires presented by the patient.

Explanation of benefit language sometimes seems to be the potential problem when LEAT provisions are applied. Most EOBs will state that a less expensive treatment could have been performed. It may be clearer to patients if the EOB could simply state what benefit the plan will allow. This difference may seem subtle, but patients sometimes misinterpret the wording "could have been performed" to mean "should

(Continued on p.163)

Dental benefits industry perspective *(Continued from p.160)*

adjudicate benefits according to the parameters of a particular employer group contract. This provision is not relevant to a dental health maintenance organization.

From a consumer's perspective, when a particular procedure is not covered in a dental benefit plan, this provision allows some portion of the treatment cost to be paid. Under this provision the dental plan will pay the allowed cost for the Least Expensive Alternative Treatment. The dentist is then able to charge the patient the difference between that service and the one actually performed.

When applying this provision a carrier is not disputing the treatment provided by the dentist; the carrier is simply applying the coverage provided by the policy to the therapy delivered to the patient to provide some level of coverage. The dental insurance industry processes more than 250 million claims annually with about 70 percent being auto-adjudicated, which means processed with computerized decision logic that is linked to the provisions of an employer's group policy. In most instances the application of a LEAT provision is done through carriers' auto-adjudication systems. Thus, the decision is not made by an individual who could be identified for the dentist as suggested by the ADA policy statement. However, there are always professional relations and customer service staff available to both dentists and consumers if a question about the application of LEAT, which is related to what is covered and not whether the treatment is appropriate.

Without this coverage provision, when a treatment is provided that is not covered, such as a posterior resin-based composite restoration, the consumer would have no coverage. Many carriers indicate that a total denial of a procedure is often more harmful to the doctor-patient relationship than the application of the LEAT benefit.

The coverage, costs and provisions of the dental benefit plan are clearly explained to employers who offer group coverage and then to the consumers that enroll in the coverage. Carriers are required by state law to provide benefit booklets and often make this information available online through printed material and accessible through customer service centers. Consumers may not, however, review these materials. Carriers agree that when alternate benefits are applied, the EOBs should indicate that the treatment provided was paid under the terms of the LEAT or alternate benefit provision of the policy. As well, dentists should also inform patients of the potential for the application of LEAT when there are a range of alternative, effective treatment options for the procedure being performed.

(Continued on p.164)

Dentist perspective *(Continued from p. 161)*

have been performed." Regarding LEAT provisions, ADA policy also states "plans which contain this clause should make the limitations of this clause understood to the plan purchaser and the dental patient." The burden of explaining LEAT provisions in an EOB, in the least misleading manner possible, should be shared by the dental plan.

The risks and benefits of all treatment alternatives should be discussed with patients and understood to achieve informed consent. Ultimately, treatment decisions are made by the patient with cost as an important consideration. If dentists explain all aspects of proposed treatment, issues with LEAT provisions can be minimized.

Dentists may want to save a copy of this article to present to patients who struggle to understand the nuances of LEAT. ■

Dental benefits industry perspective *(Continued from p.162)*

One of the most common examples of alternate benefit is the use of composite rather than amalgam restorations on posterior teeth. When a D2394 (resin-based composite restoration) is performed on a posterior tooth, the computerized logic in payment systems will apply the reimbursement for an amalgam restoration (D2161) to that tooth. The patient should be informed that their cost for treatment is the copayment on the amalgam procedure plus the cost of the difference between the two procedures. The following is an example of how the alternate benefit would be paid under some dental benefit plans:

- Dentist performs posterior resin-based composite restoration (D2394).

- Dental plan covers only amalgam restorations for posterior teeth and has an alternate benefit provision.

- Dental plan pays 80 percent of the allowable fee ($60) for (D2161) which is $48; patient pays $12 copayment.

- Patient pays difference between the allowable fee ($90) for D2394 and the $60 fee for D2161, which is $30.

- Patient total =$42; Plan total =$48.

- Total received by dentist=$90, which is full D2394 negotiated fee.

Tips: When several procedures are available to address a patient's dental needs, dentists should advise the patient that a LEAT provision may impact their out-of-pocket costs.

Dentists can submit a pre-estimate to clarify out-of-pocket costs for the consumer if needed.

Provision of a detailed informed consent with procedure cost and estimated out-of-pocket patient responsibility may also be helpful.

Carriers should review EOB language to assure that it minimizes consumer confusion with regard to benefits payments that result from application of LEAT provisions. ∎

Part 7
February 04, 2008

ADA/NADP share views on overpayment/refunds requests

This is the seventh installment of a series of *ADA News* articles on dentists' "Top Ten" concerns submitted to the ADA about dental claims. These articles include perspectives from ADA members, National Association of Dental Plans members and the Council on Dental Benefit Programs.

Past *ADA News* issues included articles on claims processing delays, dental claims denials, least expensive alternative treatment clause, and bundling and downcoding.

Subsequent articles will feature the remaining "Top Ten" concerns, which include post utilization review, assignments to participating doctors and others.

Dental benefits industry perspective

Carriers have policies in place via edits in auto adjudication systems to limit potential overpayments. However, overpayments requiring a refund can still occur for several reasons largely beyond the control of the carrier.

One of the most common reasons for refund requests is when an employer terminates a patient's dental benefits but delays notifying the carrier of this change in the employee's status. This can occur for any number of reasons, the most usual being a change of employment.

If the payer does not receive timely notice of this type of change or elimination of benefit, claims can be paid inappropriately for patients who in effect were not covered on the date of service. Once the payer learns of such a change, premiums collected by the carrier are returned because contractually, the patient bears the financial responsibility for the services rendered.

Carriers generally issue a request for refunds as soon as they become aware of an overpayment. However, events and state laws often conspire to further delay when the carrier can legally request the refund – a circumstance that forces the process to take far longer than anyone would like.

For instance, overpayments often occur when an employer decides to terminate a group contract with a carrier, and rather than notify the carrier, the employer simply fails to remit the premium. In these instances, state laws often mandate grace periods during which coverage must remain active. These grace periods are typically for 30 to 60 days during which time carriers cannot withhold claims payment nor communicate that the coverage could become suspended due to nonpayment of premium. The patient is ultimately responsible for claims under these circumstances.

Once the grace period has lapsed, or if the employer provides notification that they have elected to drop coverage or change carriers, state law requires that the termination must be retroactive to the last day the premium was paid. As a result, claims that were processed and paid during the grace period are not valid because the patients did not have effective coverage with the carrier during that time.

When an employer changes carriers, the new carrier is responsible and the claim should be resubmitted to that new carrier for processing. The patient is responsible for notifying the dentist of any change in their dental benefits; ultimately the patient should be held liable for any claims paid during this period. *(Continued on p.168)*

Dentist perspective

Many times when a third-party payer mistakenly pays a dental provider, the payer will request a refund of the overpaid amount. In some cases, refund requests have been sent to dentists more than two years after the payment was made. The patient may no longer be a patient of record with that dentist.

In most instances, the overpaid amount is deducted from future benefits paid to the dentist. In some cases, overpayments made to other dentists for the same patient may be deducted from future benefits payments to the dentist. Many members question the fairness of this practice.

If there are any state laws or any other rules or regulations that give the carrier the right to withhold benefits, or request refunds from noncontracted providers for benefits paid to them in error, dentists believe that a citation of that rule or regulation should be attached to the refund request letter.

Dental benefits industry perspective *(Continued from p.166)*

Another reason for refund requests is when a claim is submitted with an incorrect provider name or a generic practice name. This can, for example, cause an in-network claim to be paid out of network. Usually the patient or the dentist will call to inquire why the claim was paid incorrectly, prompting the carrier to reprocess the claim with the appropriate benefit.

Incorrect use of the Code on Dental Procedure and Nomenclature is another common issue in refund cases. If an incorrect CDT code is submitted that does not reflect the actual service provided by the dentist, a greater benefit may be paid inappropriately. If attention is brought to the payer – usually by a second dental office to which the patient has transferred – and the proper CDT code is applied, the claim will be reprocessed and any overpayment will be requested as a refund from the first office. Additionally, procedures are sometimes submitted for reimbursement just prior to completion, crown insertion for an example, without prior notice of the transience of some patients. Should the claim be paid and the member never return for the final insertion, a refund may be requested as the covered service was never completed. The patient would be responsible for any incurred laboratory and office cost.

Most large group employers self-fund their dental benefits, meaning they contract with a carrier only for administration. In these cases, which impact 37 million of the 170 million Americans with dental benefits, the payer has a fiduciary responsibility as well as a contractual obligation to ensure all claims are paid according to the employers' contract terms. These self-funded employers, with full expectation that a refund will be obtained and funds returned to the employer, scrutinize overpayments.

Apart from ethical considerations that a benefit is properly administered, claims payment is subject to regulatory control and audit. Payers must be able to provide documented rationale for each claim processed to state and federal regulators. Most payers will make a written request for a refund before implementing an automatic deduction from a subsequent payment.

There is no statute of limitation with respect to refund requests; however, most payers will try to request a refund as soon as an overpayment is discovered. Requests for overpayments are usually defined within a network provider agreement. With the exception of Ohio and Florida, plans are not allowed to implement automatic deductions from subsequent payment for noncontracted providers. ■

ADA/NADP share views on coordination of benefits

This is the eighth installment of a series of *ADA News* articles on dentist' "Top Ten" concerns submitted to the ADA about dental claims.

These articles include perspectives from ADA members, National Association of Dental Plans members and the Council on Dental Benefit Programs.

For more information about COB, call the ADA, toll-free, or e-mail dentalbenefits@ada.org.

To read other installments in this series on dentists' concerns about dental claims visit *ADA News* Today.

The ADA receives many general information calls regarding coordination of benefits. Dentists and staff often are not aware of the coordination of benefit rules which affect the patient's benefits. Often there does not seem to be consistency in the way different carriers coordinate benefits, which can be confusing. As with all plan information, dentists believe that applicable COB provisions should be clearly defined and described in employee benefit booklets and available on carrier Web sites.

COB is governed by state insurance law when the medical or dental plan is a regulated carrier. While state insurance law can vary from state to state, most states follow a model adopted by the National Association of Insurance Commissioners. The ADA adopted Guidelines on Coordination of Benefits in Group Plans in the mid-1990s which generally follow the NAIC Model.

With the growth of employer-sponsored medical and dental plans and collectively bargained plans that operate under federal law Employee Retirement Income Security Act of 1974 plans, the variability in COB clauses has expanded. As well, a provision called non-duplication has been added to some ERISA and other plans. COB and non-duplication provisions are the focus of this article.

Dental benefits industry perspective

COB is regulated for group carriers licensed by the state, so it is largely standardized. The exceptions are for employer-sponsored and collectively bargained (labor union) plans.

ADA policy guidelines on COB are largely consistent with the most common state laws on COB. There are three main issues raised in the questions most often posed to the ADA about application of COB regulations – which carrier is primary, what fee governs the payment from the carriers and what does the dentist charge the patient? For state regulated carriers, state insurance regulations and contract law determine how these issues are handled. What follows is an overview of the National Association of Insurance Commissioner's Model Law on COB; most state laws follow this model.

Who pays first? Who pays second?

First, only group carriers are required to coordinate. So if one of the policies covering your patient is an individual policy, then it does not coordinate. Also if one of the group carriers is an employer-sponsored plan or a collectively bargained plan, it may set its own policy for coordination. Often employer sponsored plans have a nonduplication provision which states that the employer will not pay for benefits that are reimbursed by other insurance. This provision has been included in the calculation of the premium for these policies.

When carriers are licensed by the state, like most dental carriers, state COB regulations provide guidelines by which the primary carrier and secondary carrier(s) are determined. Basically this guideline follows who is insured and how they are insured.

For dependent children, some states use the gender rule rather than the birthday rule, which makes the father's coverage primary. Check your state law before submitting claims for children. When there is a disagreement between carriers as to which rule applies, the gender rule is often used.

What is paid by the carrier: Allowable expenses

Once it is determined which company is the primary carrier and which company is the secondary carrier, claims can be processed. The primary carrier pays the claims as if there is no other insurance involved. The COB law requires the secondary carrier to calculate what the benefit would have been for the claim if there were no other carrier involved, but allows the secondary carrier to deduct the amount paid on the claim by the primary carrier from its payment. The secondary carrier then

(Continued on p.172)

Dentist perspective

The ADA policy is based on a simple premise, the patient should get the maximum allowable benefit from each plan. In total the benefit should be more than that offered by any of the plans individually, but not such that the patient receives more than the total charges for the dental services received.

Increasingly, the ADA receives calls from dentists that indicate the secondary carrier refused any additional payment because it had the same benefit level as the primary carrier. These calls refer to a nonduplication provision in the policy. This provision seems unfair to the patient that paid two premiums for coverage but received no benefit from the second premium. ADA policy opposes nonduplication provisions and at least one state, California, has enacted legislation prohibiting such provisions.

It is also hard to find a consistent pattern in which carrier is primary and secondary. This is something the dentist has to determine because the secondary carrier requires an EOB from the primary carrier to process a claim. How can dentists get a consistent picture of who to go to first? ADA policy outlines the following steps in determining a primary carrier.

- The plan covering the patient, other than as a dependent, is the primary plan.

- When both plans cover the patient as a dependent child, the plan of the parent whose birthday occurs first in a calendar year should be considered as primary.

- When a determination cannot be made in accordance with the above, the plan that has covered the patient for the longer time should be considered as primary.

- When one of the plans is a medical plan and the other is a dental plan, and a determination cannot be made in accordance with the above, the medical plan should be considered as primary.

There is also confusion when the carriers covering a patient provide different types of coverage—a capitation plan, a reduced fee plan and a full fee plan. Which fee is the charge to the patient based on? ADA policy states that dental offices should submit their usual fee, defined by ADA policy as "the fee which an individual dentist most frequently charges for a specific dental procedure," to a dental benefit plan. The benefit plan will adjudicate the claim based on its allowed fee schedules.

The Council on Dental Benefit Programs believes that if COB were standardized dentists could better estimate the appropriate reimbursement.. ■

Dental benefits industry perspective *(Continued from p.170)*

pays the claim up to 100 percent of the allowable expense if the benefit contained in the policy is great enough. So, if the dentist's charge for a procedure is $100, but the allowable expense is $80, the claim will be paid based on $80 being the maximum that can be paid.

There are two exceptions to this general rule. First, if the primary carrier is a dental health maintenance organization and the patient does not use a DHMO provider, the secondary carrier must pay the claim as if it were a primary carrier. As well, self-funded and collectively bargained employer groups operate under federal law and do not have to follow state COB laws. These groups often utilize nonduplication provisions to lower premiums. These provisions provide that the insurer will not pay for benefits that are reimbursed by other insurance. Where these provisions are present in the patient's policy, there may not be any payment from the secondary carrier.

An allowable expense is defined as the usual and customary or maximum allowable expense for the dental service when the item is covered at least in part under any of the plans involved. When a covered person is covered by two or more carriers which determine benefits on the basis of usual and customary fees or maximum allowable expense, any amount in excess of the highest usual and customary or maximum allowable is not an allowable expense. When a covered person is covered by two or more carriers, which determine benefits on the basis of contracted fees, any fee in excess of the highest contracted fee is not an allowable expense.

What to charge the patient?
Coordination of benefits can be a win-win for both patients and dental practices. Patients with more than one dental benefits program from state licensed carriers are likely to visit their dentists more frequently, knowing all or at least a large majority of treatment costs will be covered by the combination of two programs. Out-of-pocket expenses for more complex and expensive procedures are reduced or sometimes even eliminated. And dental practices can receive payment in full for all treatment rendered when reimbursement from both plans is settled.

However, COB can be complicated and time consuming for both dental practices and insurance carriers. Based on inquiries to the ADA, one of the most confusing steps in a COB situation is: "What to charge the patient?" To begin, here are two general guidelines to determine what to charge the patient:

(1) Regardless of the COB situation, always submit the fees charged to the patient as submitted charges on claim forms. (Note: Discount plans are not subject to COB

(Continued on p 174)

Dentist perspective

(See page 171)

Dental benefits industry perspective *(Continued from p.172)*

laws and regulations as they are not insurance products.) If this is not the usual fee but is discounted, include a statement regarding the discount provided. When processing the claims, the plan administrators will apply plan allowances.

(2) The participating network contractual relationship with the patient's primary plan determines the amount that can be collected from the patient. If the primary carrier has no participating network contract with your office, and the secondary carrier does, then the network relationship with the secondary carrier determines the charges to the patient. ■

Part 9
July 16, 2008

ADA/NADP share views on provider contract issues

This is the ninth installment of a series of *ADA News* articles on dentists' "Top 10" concerns submitted to the ADA about dental claims.

These articles include perspectives from ADA members, National Association of Dental Plans members and the Council on Dental Benefit Programs.

Past *ADA News* issues included articles on overpayment/refund requests, coordination of benefits, dental claims denials, bundling and downcoding and more.

Subsequent articles will feature the remaining "Top 10" concerns, which include assignment of benefits to participating dentists and post-utilization review.

Dental benefits industry perspective

Guidelines on the dentist's obligations, including processing policies (where applicable) and procedures can be found and downloaded from most insurance carrier and discount plan dentist Web sites in the form of provider reference manuals, frequently asked questions and, in many cases, under the specific claims submission guidelines sections of these Web sites. In addition, many payers include provider reference manuals as part of the welcome packets that are mailed to each new dentist. Face-to-face new dental office orientation and training sessions are usually conducted and meetings are provided upon request so that a plan's professional relations representative can visit the office to explain dental preferred provider organization, dental health maintenance organization or discount dental plan policies and procedures in greater detail.

Dentists may also view specific claims attachment requirements for all payers by accessing FastLook, a Web site service made available through the National Electronic Attachment Inc., in partnership with the National Association of Dental Plans. This portal provides one central location for dentists or their offices to search by insurance company name and Code on Dental Procedure and Nomenclature code for specific attachment requirements. ∎

Dentist perspective

If a dentist has contracted with a third-party payer, he or she may have agreed to abide by the carrier's processing policies. Often dentists may not be aware of these policies and procedures, and sometimes, the payer may not release detailed information related to the carrier's policies and procedures until the dentist becomes a participating provider. This, of course, may make it difficult for the dentist to have a clear understanding of his or her contractual obligations.. ■

Dental benefits industry perspective – component procedures:

An important feature of dental benefits for the patient is reducing out-of-pocket expenses. Along with lower copayments when using contracted providers, prohibitions on balance billing—including billing for components of a service separately – are an important part of establishing some predictability in patients' costs. Ultimately, the provisions of an employer's group policy govern what the carrier pays. If covered, the carrier may establish policies that govern payment for services that do not conflict with Health Insurance Portability and Accountability Act requirements to use the current version of the Code.

When a contracted dentist bills a patient for a procedure considered to be a component of another procedure and it is processed as one procedure, in most cases the payer is attempting to follow guidelines established in the Code.

However, in self-funded situations, employers determine covered benefits and how they are paid. These employer groups are regulated under federal law—the Employee Retirement Income Security Act of 1974—and are exempt from other requirements. About 37 million of the 170 million Americans enrolled in dental plans are covered under employer self-funded groups. This is 26 percent of the private market for dental benefits. In these cases, the payer performs as a dental administrator and is obligated by contract to process claims as the employer group specifies.

It is important to note that the Code is mandated under HIPAA as the standard procedure set and payers are legally bound to process claims based on the Code. All claims, whether submitted on a HIPAA standard electronic dental transaction or on paper, must use the dental procedure code from the version of the Code in effect on the date of service.

A variety of combinations of dental services not consistent with the Code are submitted to payers, such as pins reported separate from core build ups; adhesives, bases or liners as separate from restorations; X-rays taken during root canal therapy as a separate service from the root canal. Payers administer these component services as part of the main procedure in accordance with the Code and/or the employer's specific policy and pay benefits accordingly. (See the article on bundling and downcoding which is part of this series on dentists' concerns about dental claims originally published in the June 18, 2007 *ADA News*.

Because the patient pays for the procedure at the time services are rendered, this concern does not apply to a DDP. *(Continued on p.180)*

Dentist perspective

One of the most common complaints received from contracted dentists is an inability to bill patients for procedures that are considered by the payer to be a component of another procedure, or procedures that are disallowed or even denied by the plan. In such cases, dentists feel that they are providing free services to patients. This is especially true if the plan considers the entire procedure to be unnecessary or disallowed. Therefore, it is important for dentists to evaluate and understand contract provisions while considering a contract with a plan. For example, dentists may wish to research whether a contract provision that considers a procedure to be a component of another procedure is actually due to guidelines established in the Code. ∎

Dental benefits industry perspective—denied procedures:

(Continued from p.178)

DPPO: Since dental benefits are market-driven, coverage for certain dental procedures varies based on the group policy selected by the employer. Limitations in an employer's group policy may result in noncovered procedures or denial. The dentist may resubmit the claim with a request for review by a dental consultant if he/she feels the claim was incorrectly disallowed or denied. The employer's group policy ultimately determines what is covered. It's important for participating network dentists to note, and at times to communicate with their insured patients, that a denied claim does not necessarily mean the service wasn't necessary or beneficial. It simply means that that procedure wasn't a covered benefit. Plan communications to patients should indicate when a procedure is not covered under their plan and not imply that the procedure was unnecessary.

When a coded procedure or service is not covered by the group or individual policy, the dentist's contract with the payer determines whether the patient is billed at a contracted rate or the dentist's usual and customary fee. Some payers include a clause in their contracts with dentists that require the dentist to offer a percentage discount on noncovered procedures to the patient. This gives the patient an option to choose treatment they may not ordinarily have chosen due to financial limitations.

Most DHMOs have a provision in their agreements that address noncovered services. The participating dentist agrees to look to the patient for complete payment of noncovered dental services. ∎

Dentist perspective

(See page 179)

Dental benefits industry perspective

Business relationships are dynamic and complex in a competitive, fast-moving market for dental benefits. Some states require that carriers operate under a separate company in their state. Thus, it is not unusual for a carrier to have multiple affiliates and subsidiaries. As well, to service a particular employer group in states where a carrier may not operate, agreements may be entered into for another carrier to administer the group policy. All these arrangements to meet the demands of the market cannot be specifically anticipated and spelled out in detail when contracts are signed. Therefore, where applicable provisions exist in carrier contracts that refer generally to affiliated carriers.

However, most carriers work to proactively communicate relationships that develop rather than just rely on a clause in the contract. Some plans do this through opt-in or opt-out provisions for such arrangements. Despite these arrangements, gaps in understanding of the obligation to affiliated carriers do occur. For DPPOs and DDPs, disclosing partnerships or reciprocal network sharing arrangements is a regulatory requirement in many states. For this reason, most insurance carriers include this clause in their dentist agreement, with many listing the specific names of the affiliated and/or subsidiary carriers.

Dental carriers may use additional methods to address this issue—such as FAQ sheets included in the application packet materials or FAQs posted on their dentist Web site. These are usually accessible prior to joining a DPPO or DDP network.

Affiliation and reciprocal agreements are a rare occurrence with DHMOs. ■

Dentist perspective

Another issue that comes up frequently is the all affiliated carriers clause in many contracts. In cases where a dentist signs a contract with a plan that includes an all affiliated carriers clause, the dentist becomes a participating provider for the affiliated carrier, even if the dentist never directly contracted with the affiliated carrier. Situations such as this highlight the importance of dentists carefully reviewing their participating dentist contracts and all related materials (such as provider manuals and quality assurance and utilization plans), prior to entering into such contracts. In addition, prior to entering into such contracts, dentists would be prudent to contact the plan with which they may contract to discuss whether the contract requires them to see patients of affiliated carriers as well as any other issues related to the contract that need clarification. ■

Dental benefits industry perspective

If a contracted dentist no longer wishes to participate in DPPO, DHMO or DDP networks, carriers request that he or she submit the request in writing. Some carriers require the termination letter be mailed by certified mail, faxed, e-mailed or sent by a nationally recognized delivery service. Often there is a contractual waiting period (30, 60 or 90 days) before terminations take effect. In many states these time frames are set by law and a dentist's name will not be removed until the waiting period has elapsed.

Carriers confirm receipt of the dentist's request, as well as the termination effective date by mail or as dictated by the terms of the agreement and state law. The dentist should be removed from the Web site once notification has been received from the contracted dentist and any required waiting periods have elapsed.

Carriers are moving to electronic rather than printed directories to provide for easier updates. Employers may maintain and distribute outdated copies of provider directories without the carrier's knowledge. However, ultimately the insurance carriers bear the responsibility of updating their systems to reflect this change in status. It is important for dentists to notify carriers when they have not been removed from network listing as these systems may be outsourced or have failures that are not otherwise identified. An outdated database of participating dentists may result in the issuance of claims discrepancy notices and necessitate the reprocessing of claims, neither of which an insurance carrier desires. ■

Dentist perspective

A dentist's "participating" status is another issue. Often carriers are slow in removing a dentist from the participating status list after the dentist has terminated a carrier's contract. Dentists would be wise to submit a request in writing for carriers to remove their names from any participating provider list at the time the contract is terminated, and follow up with carriers who fail to remove a dentist's name in a timely fashion. ■

Dental benefits industry perspective

Representatives of an insurance carrier's customer relations and/or the provider relations departments may answer questions about a dentist's contract.

Questions about policy issues are best answered by a customer relations representative. The majority of carriers include customer relations phone numbers in a variety of materials and methods: the dentist Web site, provider reference guides, explanation of benefits (EOBs), application packet materials. Customer relations representatives operate from a common base of policies and procedures so responses are consistent. Assigning a specific customer service or claims representative with personal phone number could unduly burden one individual and could result in the inability to provide all dentists with the most responsive level of service.

However, many carriers assign an individual provider relations representative to dentists in a specific geographic region, as a personal plan resource and contact for dentists. This field representative interacts with customer service, claims processors and dental consultants to assist in resolving a dentist's concerns when necessary.

Some carriers' claims departments are structured to include a coordinator of dental consultant review, who works directly with the dental consultants and answers any specific questions from the dentist. Dental consultants for some carriers are also accessible for further discussion if necessary. Most of these consultants return calls in one or two business days to allow time for a thorough review of the issue or claim that is submitted.

This would not apply to discount dental plans since they do not pay claims. ■

Dentist perspective

Another common complaint among dentists is that they do not have a specific phone number for a provider service representative who could assist them with contract or policy issues. In addition, many dentists have indicated that carriers will not provide access to dental consultants for them when they have a disagreement with a consultant's assessment. ■

ADA/NADP share views on assignment of benefits

In this installment of a series on dentists' "Top Ten" concerns submitted to the ADA about dental claims, Delta Dental Plans Association joins the National Association of Dental Plans to provide the dental benefits industry perspective on assignment of benefits to participating dentists only. ADA members and the Council on Dental Benefit Programs provide the dentist perspective.

ASSIGNMENT OF BENEFITS TO PARTICIPATING DENTISTS ONLY

Dental benefits industry perspective

About 96 percent of today's dental benefits marketplace is provided under group contracts – largely through employers. Most large group employers self-fund their dental benefits, meaning they contract with a carrier only for administration of the benefits that the employer provides. These groups are regulated under federal law – Employee Retirement Income Security Act of 1974 – not state law and set their own rules with regard to assignment. In these cases, which impact 37 million of the 170 million Americans with dental benefits, the payer has a fiduciary responsibility as well as a contractual obligation to pay claims according to the employers' contract terms.

State-regulated carriers serve the balance of the market. These carriers are regulated under statutes which vary from state to state. The licensing laws and related statutes, along with their business approach to meeting the needs of a diverse employer market, influence a carrier's operational policies.

State laws requiring assignment of benefits apply to all carriers. In states where such requirements do not exist, many carriers usually honor assignment of benefits to nonparticipating dentists as a courtesy to their enrollees and to maintain consistency in their procedures state-to-state. Most of these carriers also provide a copy of the explanation of benefits to a nonparticipating dentist when he or she submits the claim on behalf of the enrollee. However, the patient's assignment of benefits and communication of that assignment through the claim form does not legally supersede the group contract. The claim form is a method of communicating information, not a legal obligation.

Some companies, usually those organized as Delta Dental member companies, approach assignment of benefits differently. With 250 million claims processed annually, almost 60 percent by paper, dentists who are not contracted must be entered into claims payment systems and are generally not familiar with carrier claim processing policies. Carriers who do not typically honor assignment of

(Continued on p.190)

Dentist perspective

Some third-party payers will only assign benefits to participating providers, even when the patients sign the appropriate assignment of benefits box on the claim form. This is a particularly damaging practice because dentists charge the patient only what will not be covered by insurance at the time of service, when assignment of benefits has been obtained. Dentists are then placed in a difficult collections position because in some cases their patients will not pay them after receiving payment from the insurance carrier.

Often the dentist will not receive a copy of the explanation of benefits and has no idea of the amount paid, or even if the claim was received and processed at all. It's hard for dentists to understand why a third-party payer would not honor the assignment of benefits from the plan participant. any dentists feel that not honoring patients' requests to assign benefits to nonparticipating providers is an attempt by carriers to get these providers to join their networks. entists believe that third-party payers that will not assign benefits to nonparticipating dentists should inform dentists of this policy upfront so that dental offices may collect money from patients at the time of treatment. ■

Dental benefits industry perspective *(Continued from p.188)*

benefits view direct payment as a value of network participation and a method of reinforcing patient selection of dentists within the established dentist network to optimize the amount of care patients can obtain under their annual maximum.

Carriers have a responsibility to inform patients of their obligations when using dentists who are not in their networks. Dental carriers do this through informational materials regarding benefits. When provided in writing, these materials are usually regulated by state requirements for readability at a grade school level. Carriers also provide Web sites where enrollees can access their evidence of coverage, which detail their out-of-pocket responsibility to the dentist. Any carrier's practice of not accepting assignment to nonparticipating providers should be explained in these benefit materials.

Carriers also have an obligation to make their policies clear and easily accessible to dentists. Most carriers do this through dedicated provider relations call centers. Increasingly, carriers are adding online systems to provide this information to dentists within the limits of privacy and security laws. Dentists should check these sources when a patient provides coverage information and before they communicate with patients about financial responsibility and payment policies.

Through dentist contracting, carriers assume the cost of a variety of functions that ease payment and collection processes for dentists while providing the opportunity to increase their patient base. Plan design incentives encouraging enrollees to obtain care from network dentists further expand the value of contracting and the benefits available to the enrollee/patient. These incentives cover a range of operational differences, from reductions on level of reimbursement to refusal of assignment to nonparticipating dentists.

Carriers must balance the interests of their enrollees with more than 100,000 dentists in the U.S. who have chosen to contract with them and noncontracting dentists. Dentists enter into contractual arrangements for a variety of reimbursement, cost and service advantages. Extending assignment of benefits and other cost savings to noncontracted dentists can diminish these advantages for contracted dentists and is a carrier choice where it is not regulated by law.

Assignment of benefits can be superseded by federal law, applicable under state law to all carriers, honored as a courtesy to enrollees or treated as an advantage for dentists who enter into contractual relationships with carriers, including compliance with carriers' payment rules and policies. All are valid carrier choices, which differentiate their operation in the marketplace just as dental offices design their operations to capture their target market. ■

ADA/NADP share views on post-utilization review

This is the final installment of a series of *ADA News* articles on dentists' "Top 10" concerns submitted to the ADA about dental claims. The articles include perspectives from ADA members, National Association of Dental Plans members and the Council on Dental Benefit Programs.

Past *ADA News* issues included articles on overpayment/refund requests, coordination of benefits, claims processing delays, dental claims denials, least expensive alternative treatment clauses, bundling and downcoding and more.

Visit www.ada.org/goto/top10concerns to read other installments in this series.

For more information about dental benefits issues, call the ADA toll-free or e-mail dentalbenefits@ada.org.

Dental benefits industry perspective

For state licensed dental insurance carriers, utilization review is a formal process regulated by the states, not by individual carriers. State regulations apply to all health insurance and post-utilization review is common in medical claims. While states may differ in exact requirements for utilization review, most include the key provisions set in the Model Utilization Review Act adopted by the National Association of Insurance Commissioners. These include:

- written procedures which document clinical review criteria;
- mechanisms for consistent application of criteria:
    1. analytical methods utilized;
    2. time periods for conducting reviews;
- administration by qualified health care professionals;
- confidentiality;
- disclosure of the process to covered persons;
- access to review staff for both covered persons and participating providers;
- an appeals process for adverse determinations.

Utilization review is defined by the NAIC as "a set of formal techniques designed to monitor the use of or evaluate the medical necessity, appropriateness, efficacy or efficiency of health care services, procedures, or settings." The NAIC utilization review model was designed to provide safeguards for both health care providers and patients in the utilization review process.

About 96 percent of today's dental benefits marketplace is provided under group contracts—largely through employers. Most large group employers self-fund their dental benefits, meaning they contract with a carrier only for administration of the benefits that the employer provides. These groups are regulated under federal law—the Employee Retirement Income Security Act of 1974—not state law. Under ERISA, employers set their own rules with regard to administration of benefits, including utilization review. An estimated 37 million of the 170 million Americans with dental benefits are covered under these self-funded ERISA-protected programs, and about 133 million Americans are covered by carriers subject to state regulation.

In the dental market, the written procedures for utilization review are composed with input from the carrier's Dental Advisory Committee, dental director and in some instances, outside dental consultants. The process that results usually compares a dentist's practice patterns to those of peers in the community and across the nation. Most participating dentist agreements contain language that requires participation in some form of claims utilization review process.

(Continued on p.194)

Dentist perspective

The ADA is hearing from a number of dentists who are undergoing post-utilization reviews, also called retrospective claim audits.

Often these audits begin with the carrier internally monitoring use of the dentist's claims. Usually the dentist is unaware that his or her claims are being monitored.

If the carrier determines that the dentist has practice patterns that it believes warrant claims evaluation, the carrier can "flag" the dentist in its claims system. When a dentist is flagged, claims for certain procedures are reviewed. Usually the dentist is asked to submit additional documentation regarding the necessity of the procedure. Often the dentist doesn't understand why the carrier is requesting additional documentation for certain procedures.

When a dentist is flagged in the claim system for utilization review, the Council on Dental Benefit Programs recommends that a clear explanation be sent to the dentist advising of the review, what procedures are being reviewed and what specific information needs to be submitted with each claim.

The council further recommends that dentists be advised on how they can become "unflagged." In addition, dentists should be advised if the review could result in an in-office audit of the patient's charts and billing records and that potential refund requests may be pursued. If the review results in a refund request, the carrier should provide information to the dentist to enable him or her to appeal the carrier's decision. ∎

Dental benefits industry perspective *(Continued from p.192)*

Utilization review may be performed by the payer or it could be delegated to a certified utilization review organization. Carriers have written procedures for the services that are reviewed and the parameters against which they are evaluated. A utilization review program typically involves pretreatment review (i.e., predetermination of benefits) and retrospective review (i.e., post-utilization review). In this article we will concentrate on retrospective utilization review.

Carriers perform retrospective utilization review to ensure appropriateness of care for their members. It is a misconception that utilization review is done solely to control costs and limit expenses. The main focus of utilization review is to identify treatment patterns that fall outside of statistically significant parameters.

Carriers conduct utilization review by focusing on specific procedures performed by dentists, which when compared to statistically relevant data, may indicate differences in practice patterns compared to the entire dentist population from which the claims data is analyzed.

Patterns of clinical activity and evaluation of treatment outcomes are based on quantitative data obtained from claims data. This data provides information and a method of evaluating the clinical activity patterns of each provider in relation to established peer benchmarks of over- and under-utilization, upcoding, procedure splitting and other irregularities.

Based on the statistical variances noted, a dentist may be identified for prepayment review consideration. However, most carriers will only initiate this type of "review" (or "flag") if the identified statistically outlying pattern occurs over an established period (three contiguous quarters).

Usually, carriers contact the dentist or dental office to determine whether any unique aspects of the dentist's practice may explain the differences in practice pattern. If no extenuating circumstances exist and the dentist is placed on prepayment review, the carrier should provide an overview of the utilization review results as well as the process.

If the statistical variation is resolved over a designated period of time, the dentist should be removed from prepayment review. If the questionable statistical pattern is not resolved, a range of other corrective actions exist, such as in-office chart review or revocation of participating status.

Should a refund request result from the chart review, carriers' procedures provide for specific appeals processes. ∎

Part 12
December 17, 2009

ADA/NADP share views on a single claim form

Paper processing issues are among the most frequent claims problems the dental benefits industry reports to the ADA Council on Dental Benefit Programs.

The topic launches a series of *ADA News* articles about the dental benefits industry's "Top 10" concerns submitted to the ADA about dental claims processing. It follows articles published from 2006-08 examining the "Top 10" dental claims concerns that dentists reported. That series was developed in response to CDBP discussions with the National Association of Dental Plans and the payer industry to facilitate communication and eliminate claims problems for members and patients.

"In its leadership role, the ADA anticipates the needs of dentists to facilitate changes that are of maximum benefit and minimal inconvenience to a practice," says Dr. Bert Oettmeier, chair of the Council on Dental Benefit Programs.

With a goal of clarifying information necessary for the timely and consistent adjudication of claims, these articles will include perspectives from ADA members, National Association of Dental Plans members and the Council on Dental Benefit Programs about topics within three broad categories:

- paper processing issues;
- education of dental office staff;
- myths and misunderstandings.

NADP member companies represent some 80 percent of the estimated 176 million Americans covered by dental benefit plans.

This first installment features the one of three topics falling under the category of paper processing issues, the single claim form. Subsequent articles will cover the remaining "Top 10" concerns, which include information technology, how fees for services are developed and diagnoses.

Visit www.ada.org/goto/top10concerns to read other installments in this series.

For more information about dental benefits issues, call the ADA toll-free or e-mail dentalbenefits@ada.org.

Dental benefits industry perspective

One simple step to improve paper claims filing:

In 2008, 51 percent of all dental claims were submitted to dental benefits companies electronically and 49 percent of dental claims were submitted on a paper claim form. While the Health Insurance Portability and Accountability Act of 1996 mandates a standardized format for electronic claims, no such mandate exists for a standard paper dental claim form.

This lack of uniformity creates a paper dental claim processing system that is unnecessarily complex, cumbersome and costly. The situation calls for the adoption and use of a single standardized paper dental claim form—the American Dental Association Dental Claim Form.

Unnecessary Costs:

Although 49 percent of dental claims are submitted on paper, the data is typically converted to electronic formats. This conversion takes place via manual data entry or by scanning and using Optical Character Recognition. The lack of a standard dental claim form increases the costs of claims processing in both the data entry and OCR processes.

Required data is not entered in the same place on every form. Dental benefits industry staff entering the data must look in multiple locations for the same information. When a few additional seconds of staff time are multiplied by the hundreds of millions of claims processed each year, the impact to processing, staff costs and delays in reimbursement become clear.

This issue also impacts OCR processing. OCR programs can recognize and convert data from a paper form into electronic data. However, the lack of consistency in the location of information can make the data difficult to retrieve and negatively impact the efficiency of the data captured. In some cases, the data location is so skewed that the paper form is transferred to a staff member so data can be re-entered manually. This doubles the amount of time needed to compile data prior to review and adjudication.

Paper chase:

Affiliated Network Services, one of the larger clearinghouses for dental claims, reports almost 50 different claim formats can be received for processing in any given month.

(Continued on p.198)

Dentist perspective

The American Dental Association agrees with the underlying theme of the National Association of Dental Plans' adjoining article—adoption and use of a single standard paper dental claim form by all sectors of the dental community. Such a single standard exists: it's the ADA Dental Claim Form.

In 1991 the ADA House of Delegates formally recognized the value of a standard claim form to dentists, third-party payers and other sectors of the dental community by adopting policy entitled ADA's Dental Claim Form. This policy, which continues in force today, states that the ADA urges universal use and acceptance of this form, as well as the Code on Dental Procedures and Nomenclature, for claim submission.

The ADA recommends that dentists use the most recent version of the ADA Dental Claim Form, while also acknowledging that use of the ADA claim form is voluntary. The form's current version is in widespread use. Member dentists inform ADA staff that many third-party payers providing coverage to patients require use of the current version of the ADA Dental Claim Form as a result of the payers' own business practices or through provisions in participating provider contracts. Some state Medicaid agencies also mandate use of the ADA's claim form for reporting services provided to covered individuals.

Linking the paper and electronic claim, and automated processing:
The paper ADA Dental Claim Form's data content served as the starting point for creation of an electronic dental claim format by ANSI ASC X12.

ANSI ASC X12 is the acronym that stands for American National Standards Institute Accredited Standards Committee X12. X12 is the specific accredited committee that develops electronic data interchange standards and related documents for various sectors of the business community, including health care. X12N is the subcommittee responsible for development of insurance EDI standards. Several X12 transactions have been named as Health Insurance Portability and Accountability Act of 1996 standards. X12 work led to the HIPAA standard electronic dental claim transaction – a federal requirement for all health care providers filing electronic transactions.

In 2001 the ADA House of Delegates recognized that HIPAA standards can also influence the ADA Dental Claim Form. ADA policy adopted that year stated that paper form data content should be coordinated with the HIPAA standard electronic dental claim transaction. Such content coordination is evident in the current version (2006 © American Dental Association), which incorporates changes that enable reporting of the national provider identifier, also required under the Health Insurance Portability and Accountability Act of 1996. *(Continued on p.199)*

Dental benefits industry perspective *(Continued from p.196)*

Why so many different claim forms? In some cases, providers submit old, outdated forms to use up a stockpile they may have purchased. While this may seem to be an efficient use of office inventory, this "efficiency" actually impedes the timely processing of claims. It's the same as using old letterhead after a move to use up stock when it would actually increase confusion and cause delays.

Still other claim forms can be generated as printouts from practice management systems dental offices use. The three most widely-used practice management software systems have the ability to produce the current paper ADA Dental Claim Form. However, many providers have not updated the software and the printouts are in outdated formats. What appears to be a savings by not updating the software can actually slow down the processing of outdated formats as they end up being manually processed.

In other cases, a large employer may request a dental plan administrator to customize a claim form to brand the employee benefit programs. This is similar to customization requested by self-administered plans such as labor unions. Brand marketing may seem logical at first, but this customization actually leads to delays in claim processing.

The additional cost and complexity added to the claims processing system by the use of outdated, nonstandard or personalized claims forms supports the use of a single standardized dental claim form across the dental industry.

Simple solution:
Education is key in helping those in the dental industry see how a simple solution can quickly and easily reduce the unnecessary costs involved with processing claims and expedite payment to providers.

While the complete solution is to move to processing claims via electronic data interchange, the second best option is to adopt, implement and use the ADA Dental Claim Form for all dental paper claims. If there is only one standardized dental claim form, dental office staff members do not have to coordinate claim forms with different dental plans. When filing secondary insurance, coordination of benefits would be made easier as office staff and benefit plans would have a consistent data format to compare coverage.

(Continued on p.200)

Dentist perspective *(Continued from p.197)*

NADP's adjoining article also notes that use of a standard paper form brings a variety of preparation and processing efficiencies, with particular mention of automated data entry via Optical Character Recognition technology used by third-party payers. A red ink form that supports OCR has been and continues to be offered in the ADA Catalog (J404).

Updating the ADA Dental Claim Form:

The ADA Council on Dental Benefit Programs has ADA Bylaws responsibility for the ADA Dental Claim Form. This responsibility includes determining content and format, as well as when a new version of the form should be introduced. The council considers suggested changes from several sources including dentists, practice staff and individual council members as representatives of their district's dentists.

In addition, the council established the Dental Claim Form Advisory Committee to engage varied sectors of the dental community in discussion of possible changes to the ADA Dental Claim Form. As an advisory body, DeCFAC offers suggestions for form changes on its own, as well as commenting on changes suggested by others in the dental community. DeCFAC is comprised of representatives from the Council on Dental Benefit Programs and the Council on Dental Practice, representatives from third-party payer organizations, including NADP, and electronic data interchange agencies.

Education:

The ADA uses several different avenues to promote adoption and correct use of the ADA Dental Claim Form. A separate section of the CDT manual contains comprehensive claim form completion instructions. This feature, first seen in CDT-2005, provides field-by-field guidance on form completion for dentists, front-office staff and practice management system vendors using software that prints the claim form. The instructions are illustrated with the relevant portion of the form, and include codes (area of the oral cavity, tooth number, provider specialty) that are used when preparing a claim form. These codes are the same codes that are used in the HIPAA standard electronic dental claim transaction – another example of the march toward standard data content.

(Continued on p.201)

Dental benefits industry perspective *(Continued from p.198)*

Utilizing the readily and easily available ADA Dental Claim Form can:

- increase consistency;
- increase claims processing speed;
- reduce the potential for human error;
- streamline the process;
- reduce costs.

In one simple step, providers and dental offices can move toward a more efficient and productive paper claims processing system to benefit everyone involved in the process.

NADP encourages the adoption of the ADA Dental Claim Form as the single standardized paper claim form for all aspects of the dental benefits industry to increase efficiency and efficacy while reducing confusion and costs. ∎

Dentist perspective *(Continued from p.199)*

Additional information on claim form use and completion is found in the CDT 2009-2010 Question & Answer section, the CDT Companion and the council's half-day Code Workshop presentation. Council staff provides information about the form to dentists, office staff, third-party payers, practice management system vendors and government agencies that write or call with questions.

Future:

When will the need for a paper claim form end? Will there always be an ADA Dental Claim Form? Despite continuing progress toward a paper-free, or at least a paper-limited dental practice, there is no set timetable for such goals. For the foreseeable future, the ADA Dental Claim Form fulfills the need for a standard paper dental claim format. ■

Claim Rejection – Payer
Misuse of the *Code* or
Something Else?

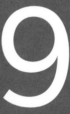

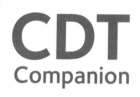

Chapter 9
Claim Rejection – Payer Misuse of the *Code* or Something Else?

Introduction

Some claims will be rejected by a third-party payer and the reason for denial helps determine what should be done next. This section of *The CDT Companion* contains information that will help you determine what to do – information about how the *Code* may be used by a payer; how to avoid misconceptions on what may be improper use, and who to contact when issues with payers arise.

"The existence of a dental procedure code does not mean that the procedure is a covered or reimbursed benefit…" is a quote from the preface of the first (1990) and every later edition of the CDT manual. This is an important concept as available coverage is determined by dental benefit plan design. Plan limitations and exclusions vary, which means a procedure that is covered by one patient's benefit plan may not be covered by another patient's plan. Implants are one example of procedures that are not covered by all plans.

One Common Misconception – HIPAA

Under HIPAA (Health Insurance Portability and Accountability Act of 1996) the *Code on Dental Procedures and Nomenclature (Code)* was named as the federal standard for reporting dental procedures on electronic dental claims. Some have interpreted this to mean that since the *Code* is a national standard, payers must provide reimbursement for any valid procedure code reported on a claim. This interpretation goes beyond what the HIPAA regulations say.

The regulations say four things:

1. A standard electronic dental claim may only contain procedures found in the *Code*

2. A dentist must submit the procedure code that is valid on the date of service

3. A payer may not refuse to accept for processing a claim with a valid procedure code

4. A payer's benefit plan design and adjudication policies apply when processing a claim

In other words HIPAA establishes a standard for communicating information about services provided to a patient. HIPAA does not influence a payer's claim adjudication process (e.g., application of policies and benefit limitations & exclusions). The CDT manual's preface statement (above) and HIPAA are consistent.

The ADA's Viewpoint

Third-party issues continue to concern members, in particular as they relate to the appropriate use of the *Code*. *Code* misuse takes on a number of different forms and the ways misuse can be addressed by the ADA need to be better understood.

The *Code* is a copyrighted work owned by the ADA and is licensed for use to outside entities. The copyright license does not control the manner in which the *Code* is used for internal claims adjudication, but prohibits changing the actual verbiage of the *Code*. Unlicensed use of the *Code* is aggressively pursued by the ADA's Division of Legal Affairs.

Potential appropriate uses of the *Code* that may be inadvertently perceived as misuse include:

- When a third-party adjudicates a claim based on a least expensive alternative treatment clause in an agreement with a plan purchaser and changes the submitted procedure code to another procedure code, there is no misuse of the *Code* if the claim is properly adjudicated under the terms of the benefit plan agreement.

- When a third-party denies a claim based on frequency limitations after changing the submitted procedure code to another procedure code, there is no misuse of the *Code* if the claim is properly adjudicated under the terms of the benefit plan agreement. One example of this, under proper circumstances, might be the changing of a minimal number of periapical radiographs and bitewings to a complete series and then denying the benefit due to frequency limitations for a complete series.

An illustration of how the ADA tries to remedy these issues is that the ADA was successful in obtaining a change to the *Code,* effective January 1, 2009, that adds a descriptor defining a complete series. This should assist in working with payers to define benefits appropriately, but it does not prevent payers from designing benefit plans that may alternatively benefit to another procedure.

What constitutes potential Payer misuse of the Code?

Insurance carriers will adjudicate claims based on agreements they have in force with plan purchasers (generally employers or union groups). So long as the agreements meet legal muster in terms of, e.g., clarity, consistency, and compliance with applicable laws and regulations, they will not generally be susceptible to legal attack, although even with valid agreements there may be legal questions concerning interpretation and scope of language in certain instances.

For example, many of these plans have contract provisions that provide for bundling or downcoding of submitted procedure codes prior to claim adjudication. Bundling and downcoding are defined as:

Bundling of Procedures: The systematic combining of distinct dental procedure codes by third-party payers that results in a reduced benefit for the patient/ beneficiary.

Downcoding: A practice of third-party payers in which the benefit code has been changed to a less complex and/or lower cost procedure than what was reported except where delineated in contract agreements.

Under the terms of a particular contract, then, Bundling and/or Downcoding may be generally permitted. But, even if they are there is still the possibility that either one could be misused or abused by a payer in a particular instance. The challenge is to know, or at least to have an informed sense about, how to distinguish between true payer *Code* misuse and payer practices that, although perhaps obnoxious, are not legally objectionable. The ADA is here to help you in this regard.

The above comments apply equally to the discussion and examples that follow. Denial or reduction of benefits based on the benefit plan or participating provider contract terms (when applicable) are perhaps not misuse of the *Code*. There are other potential misuses of the *Code* such as:

- When a dental office submits a claim with a valid procedure code to a third-party and the third-party lists a different procedure code on the Explanation of Benefits (EOB) sent to the patient, without reference to the code originally submitted, a possible misuse of the *Code* exists.

- If a third-party does not accept a claim submitted with a valid procedure code submitted by a dental office, a possible misuse of the *Code* exists.

What Do Your Patient's Benefit Plan and Your Participating Provider Contract Say?

Dental benefit plan limitations and exclusions affect how a claim is adjudicated and, as noted above, a payer may reject or not reimburse a claim in accordance with the benefit plan's provisions. Just as benefit plan designs vary, there is variation in participating provider contract provisions, and if you have one (or more) each must be reviewed to see how claim submission and processing may be affected. The ADA Contract Analysis Service can assist members in identifying areas of provider contract agreements that may be noteworthy.

Benefit plans are contracts between the purchaser and third-party payer. The benefit plan's design is determined by payer and the purchaser, which is usually an employer that is providing coverage for the company's employees and dependents. Premium cost is a factor in determining richness of coverage. This is why some plans state that a prophylaxis for a patient through age 15 will always be based on the "child prophy" procedure code (**D1120**), or that the plan will only reimburse no more than two **D4910s** per calendar year. ADA policy on benefit plan design sees things differently, but is advisory, not regulatory.

Participating provider contracts are between the dentist and payer. These contracts may include provisions that require you to accept least expensive alternative treatment "LEAT" reimbursement, or agree to reimbursement based on Payer guidelines instead of specific procedure codes reported on a claim. A dentist who signs a participating provider contract is generally bound to its legally sound provisions. Likewise, the payer is also bound to the contract provisions and cannot obligate you to do something that is beyond the signed agreement.

Examples of what Is OK, and Is Not OK.
Bear in mind these are all hypothetical examples and each is limited to the facts given for it.

Example 1:

- OK: payer applies benefit plan limitations & exclusions – and says so

    > e.g., patient's benefit plan does not cover any restorative procedure delivered on the same day a **D4355** is reported

- Not OK: payer ignores procedure code's nomenclature or descriptor

    > e.g., payer states that diagnostic radiographs are part of the **D3310** procedure and cannot be reported separately

- Not OK: payer EOB message implies that dentist reported incorrect procedure on claim

Comments

A payer may deny a claim with valid procedure code when the denial is based on legally permissible benefit plan limitations and exclusions, or on provisions of a participating provider contract. Such denial would not be *Code* "misuse."

The Explanation of Benefit (EOB) document should make the payer's action clear, namely, that denial was based on benefit plan design and that the procedure codes reported by dentist were valid.

When the EOB does not make the payer's action clear, both the patient and dentist receive an incomplete or misleading explanation. The dentist should report this to the ADA.

Example 2:

- Not OK – you report **D1110** and payer directs the dentist to report **D1120** for reimbursement

    > Patient is 13 with full adult dentition and plan design sets 15 as adult age

    > Payer is asking the dentist to report wrong procedure to be consistent with the benefit plan design – this should be resisted and reported to the ADA

- But – OK for payer to accept **D1110** and pay at **D1120** based on plan design

Comments

In this example the payer wants the dentist to report procedures based on the benefit plan design, not the service delivered. Dentists should report procedures accurately and truthfully on the claim. When a payer states that a dentist must do otherwise, report such occurrences to the ADA.

EOB messages should note that dentist correctly reported procedure based on patient's clinical condition. There should also be a message that states claim adjudication was based on different procedure due to the benefit plan's limitations and exclusions.

Example 3:

- You report **D0120, D1120** and **D1203**

    > Payer says that these are not separate procedures

    > Payer says all three procedures are part of **D0120**

- Not OK –

    > Payer is redefining **D0120**

    > Payer may be "bundling"

        o Combining separate procedures into one so that reimbursement for covered services is reduced

Comments

This is an example of a situation that should be reported to the ADA.

Note: Some situations that appear to be bundling may not be. For example, a dentist who signed a participating provider contract may have agreed to accept single reimbursement for several procedures.

Example 4 –

- EOB to patient shows different codes

    > Claim form: **D0120** and **D1110**

    > EOB: **D0120** and **D1120**

    o Message says these are the correct codes for child patient

- Not OK: payer implication that dentist reported incorrect procedures on claim

Comments

This is an example of situation that should be reported to the ADA.

The payer's EOB should acknowledge that reimbursement was based on plan design.

Contacting the ADA

The ADA Member Service Center (MSC) is your first point of contact when you have questions about the *Code* or its use, or to report possible third-party payer *Code* "misuse." MSC staff will either answer your question immediately or refer your inquiry to the appropriate ADA agency for action. Appropriate ADA agencies include the Council on Dental Benefit Programs and the Division of Legal Affairs.

Please contact the MSC by telephone using either the toll-free number found on the ADA membership card, or by direct dial (312-440-2500).

Why contact the ADA?

Payers using the *Code* must be licensed to do so – and abide by the copyright license. Any payer actions that do not adhere to contractual obligations may represent misuse of the *Code*, and be reason to seek redress.

The copyright license does not dictate how a procedure code is to be reimbursed and cannot be used as a tool to force payers to use the *Code* in a particular manner. However, arbitrary payer action is an ADA concern. Even if an objectionable use of the *Code* is not a license violation or illegal, ADA staff remains available to contact third-party payers, attempting to discuss the issues and to resolve potential conflicts. Dentist reports of concerns enable ADA staff to address individual issues with payers, as well as providing the means to determine, monitor and address patterns of payer actions.

Dental/Medical Cross Coding

10

CDT
Companion

Chapter 10
Dental/Medical Cross Coding

Introduction

Dental claims filed with or covered by medical benefit plans are different from those filed with or covered by dental benefit plans. Filing claims with a patient's medical benefit plan can be done using the "1500" paper form or HIPAA electronic equivalent. Medical claim forms require the use of CPT® procedure codes and ICD-9-CM diagnostic codes. Various dental-to-medical (*Code*-to-CPT®) cross-coding references are available. CPT® codes are available from the American Medical Association at www.ama-assn.org.

1500 Health Insurance Claim Form

Information on the "1500" form, including completion instructions, can be found at: www.nucc.org

Much of the "1500" form content will be familiar to anyone who prepares dental claims. However the reporting of treatment procedures has some additional and less familiar requirements.

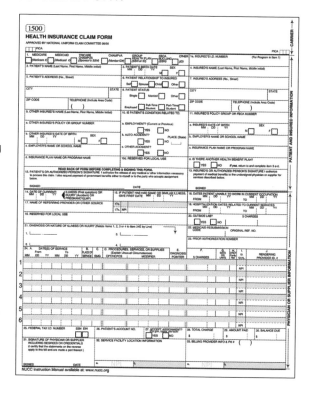

Reporting treatment begins with documenting the patient's diagnoses in box 21. The form allows up to four individual ICD-9-CM diagnosis codes to be recorded.

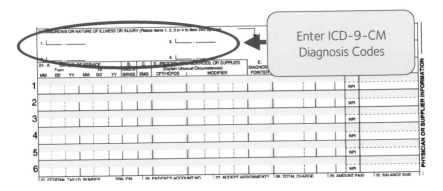

Section 24 allows up to six entries using the CPT® or HCPCS medical procedure codes corresponding to the dental treatment performed.

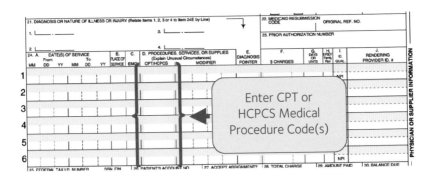

Additional details about each procedure can be reported utilizing the HCPCS modifiers and up to four modifiers can be used with each procedure. Modifiers are designated by two alphanumeric characters which are to be entered in the appropriate spaces on the form. Modifiers allow for the explanation of specific elements which may include duration, location, number of incidences, etc.

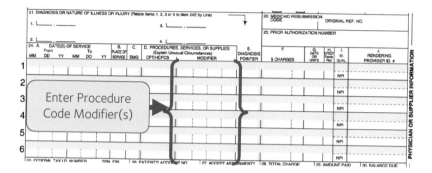

Each procedure must be tied to a diagnosis. The number, corresponding to the diagnosis listed in box 21, is recorded in column "E" for each procedure.

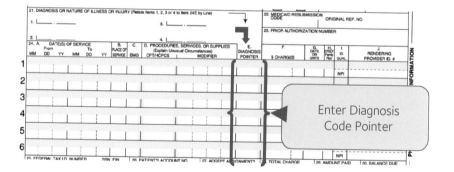

Diagnosis Codes

The International Classification of Diseases, 9th Edition, Clinical Modification (ICD-9-CM), Volumes 1 and 2 (including the official ICD-9-CM Guidelines for Coding and Reporting) as updated and distributed by the Department of Health and Human Services, is the code set used to document the following conditions:

- Diseases;
- Injuries;
- Impairments;
- Other health-related problems and their manifestations
- Causes of Injury, disease, impairment, or other health related problems.

A list of ICD-9-CM codes can be found at: www.cdc.gov/nchs/icd9.htm, which is one of several on-line sources.

Dental Caries in ICD-9-CM

> This is a sampling of the ICD-9-CM code set that may be suitable for a claim involving dental services. Diagnosis codes are available for many conditions applicable to dentistry.

521 Diseases of hard tissues of teeth
    521.0   Dental caries
    521.00 Dental caries, unspecified
    521.01 Dental caries limited to enamel
           Initial caries
           White spot lesion
    521.02 Dental caries extending into dentine
    521.03 Dental caries extending into pulp
    521.04 Arrested dental caries
    521.05 Odontoclasia
           Infantile melanodontia
           Melanodontoclasia
           Excludes:
               internal and external

Dental to Medical Coding Examples

There are a growing number of dentists who submit claims to their patients' medical benefit plans. As noted earlier in this chapter there are significant differences in how claims are prepared and submitted to a patient's medical benefit plan versus your experience in filing dental benefit plan claims.

Claims filed against a medical benefit plan use formats or codes that are not developed or maintained by the American Dental Association. Therefore the following examples of how a dental procedure could be reported as a medical benefit plan claim are advisory and intended to provide general, not definitive, guidance.

The 108 examples that follow were selected based on the nature and number of inquires for medical cross coding guidance received by ADA staff. These examples should address most of the situations a dentist may encounter when considering filing a claim against a patient's medical benefit plan.

These cross coding examples are presented as a series of tables, in a format that begins with the dental procedure code that is followed by one or more available medical procedure codes, and by one or more available medical diagnosis codes.

These examples and their solutions are not to be considered legal advice or a guarantee that individual payer contracts will follow this assistance.

Medical procedure codes come from two sources, the American Medical Association's Current Procedure Terminology (CPT) code set and the federal government's Healthcare Common Procedure Code Set (HCPCS). All medical diagnosis codes come from the federal government's International Classification of Diseases-9th Revision-Clinical Modification (ICD-9-CM) code set.

> NOTE: When selecting a medical procedure code the rule of thumb is to first look at the CPT code set to determine if there is an appropriate code to use. If there is none, a HCPCS code may be used. HCPCS codes are shown in these examples where their use might be appropriate.

There may be additional medical procedure codes and diagnosis codes than those shown in a particular table as both CPT (and HCPCS) and ICD-9-CM are larger than the *Code on Dental Procedures and Nomenclature (Code)*. For example, in 2008 CPT contained over 8,800 codes; the 2011-2012 version of the *Code* contains 592 procedure codes. This is why the tables recommend checking CPT and ICD-9-CM for other possible codes that may better reflect the service and condition being reported. You may also encounter situations where the dental procedure you wish to report is not among the examples in these tables.

Should such situations arise please contact an independent source of dental to medical procedure cross-coding information.

- Sources for medical procedure codes include, but are not limited to:

    1. American Medical Association
       http://www.ama-assn.org/ama/pub/physician-resources/solutions-managing-your-practice/coding-billing-insurance/cpt.shtml
       OR (800) 621-8335

    2. National Dental Advisory Service
       www.ndas.com OR 800-669-3337

    3. Webb Dental
       www.webbdental.com

    4. Centers for Medicare and Medicaid Services (HCPCS) –
       http://www.cms.hhs.gov/HCPCSReleaseCodeSets
       OR 877-267-2323

- Sources for medical diagnosis codes include, but are not limited to:

    1. National Center for Health Statistics
       http://www.cdc.gov/nchs/icd.htm
       or 800-232-4636

    2. icd9cm.chrisendres.com

    3. www.icd9coding.com

    4. Medical Coding Books
       http://www.medicalcodingbooks.com
       OR 866-900-8300

Please note that the dental procedure code entries in the examples that follow show the five character alphanumeric code and the applicable nomenclature. Full nomenclatures and descriptors for these entries are found in the CDT manual section that contains the *Code*.

I. Diagnostic

	Dental Procedure Code (*Code on Dental Procedures and Nomenclature*)
D0140	limited oral evaluation - problem focused
	Available Medical Procedure Code(s) – CPT **(Current Procedure Terminology)**
99201	Office or other outpatient visit for the evaluation and management of a new patient, which requires these 3 key components: • A problem focused history; • A problem focused examination; • Straightforward medical decision making. Counseling and/or coordination of care with other providers or agencies are provided consistent with the nature of the problem(s) and the patient's and/or family's needs. Usually, the presenting problem(s) are limited or minor. Physicians typically spend 10 minutes face-to-face with the patient and/or family.
99212	Office or other outpatient visit for the evaluation and management of an established patient, which requires at least 2 of these 3 key components: • A problem focused history; • A problem focused examination; • Straightforward medical decision making. Counseling and/or coordination of care with other providers or agencies are provided consistent with the nature of the problem(s) and the patient's and/or family's needs. Usually, the presenting problem(s) are limited or minor. Physicians typically spend 10 minutes face-to-face with the patient and/or family.
	See CPT (Evaluation and Management section) for additional coding options.
	Available Medical Diagnosis Code(s) - ICD-9-CM **(International Classification of Diseases-9th Revision-Clinical Modification)**
	See ICD-9-CM Section 520 - 529 (Diseases of Oral Cavity, Salivary Glands, and Jaws) for possible diagnosis codes.

Dental Procedure Code *(Code on Dental Procedures and Nomenclature)*	
D0150	comprehensive oral evaluation – new or established patient
Available Medical Procedure Code(s) – CPT (Current Procedure Terminology)	
99204	Office or other outpatient visit for the evaluation and management of a new patient, which requires these 3 key components: • A comprehensive history; • A comprehensive examination; • Medical decision making of moderate complexity. Counseling and/or coordination of care with other providers or agencies are provided consistent with the nature of the problem(s) and the patient's and/or family's needs. Usually, the presenting problem(s) are of moderate to high severity. Physicians typically spend 45 minutes face-to-face with the patient and/or family.
99215	Office or other outpatient visit for the evaluation and management of an established patient, which requires at least 2 of these 3 key components: • A comprehensive history; • A comprehensive examination; • Medical decision making of high complexity. Counseling and/or coordination of care with other providers or agencies are provided consistent with the nature of the problem(s) and the patient's and/or family's needs. Usually, the presenting problem(s) are of moderate to high severity. Physicians typically spend 40 minutes face-to-face with the patient and/or family.
	See CPT (Evaluation and Management section) for additional coding options.
Available Medical Diagnosis Code(s) – ICD-9-CM (International Classification of Diseases-9th Revision-Clinical Modification)	
	See ICD-9-CM Section 520 - 529 (Diseases of Oral Cavity, Salivary Glands, and Jaws) for possible diagnosis codes.

Dental Procedure Code
(Code on Dental Procedures and Nomenclature)

D0160	detailed and extensive oral evaluation – problem focused, by report

Available Medical Procedure Code(s) – CPT
(Current Procedure Terminology)

99213	Office or other outpatient visits for the evaluation and management of an established patient, which requires at least 2 of these 3 key components:
	• An expanded problem focused history;
	• An expanded problem focused examination;
	• Medical decision making of low complexity.
	Counseling and/or coordination of care with other providers or agencies are provided consistent with the nature of the problem(s) and the patient's and/or family's needs. Usually, the presenting problems are of low to moderate severity.
	Physicians typically spend 15 minutes face-to-face with the patient and/or family.
99214	Office or other outpatient visit for the evaluation and management of an established patient, which requires at least 2 of these 3 key components:
	• A detailed history;
	• A detailed examination;
	• Medical decision making of moderate complexity.
	Counseling and/or coordination of care with other providers or agencies are provided consistent with the nature of the problem(s) and the patient's and/or family's needs. Usually, the presenting problem(s) are of moderate to high severity.
	Physicians typically spend 25 minutes face-to-face with the patient and/or family.
	See CPT (Evaluation and Management section) for additional coding options.

Available Medical Diagnosis Code(s) – ICD-9-CM
(International Classification of Diseases-9th Revision-Clinical Modification)

	See ICD-9-CM Section 520 - 529 (Diseases of Oral Cavity, Salivary Glands, and Jaws) for possible diagnosis codes.

	Dental Procedure Code *(Code on Dental Procedures and Nomenclature)*
D0170	re-evaluation - limited, problem focused (established patient; not post-operative visit)

	Available Medical Procedure Code(s) – CPT **(Current Procedure Terminology)**
99212	Office or other outpatient visit for the evaluation and management of an established patient, which requires at least two of these three key components: • A problem focused history; • A problem focused examination; • Straightforward medical decision making. Counseling and/or coordination of care with other providers or agencies are provided consistent with the nature of the problem(s) and the patient's and/or family's needs. Usually, the presenting problem(s) are self limited or minor. Physicians typically spend 10 minutes face-to-face with the patient and/or family
99213	Office or other outpatient visits for the evaluation and management of an established patient, which requires at least 2 of these 3 key components: • An expanded problem focused history; • An expanded problem focused examination; • Medical decision making of low complexity. Counseling and/or coordination of care with other providers or agencies are provided consistent with the nature of the problem(s) and the patient's and/or family's needs. Usually, the presenting problems are of low to moderate severity. Physicians typically spend 15 minutes face-to-face with the patient and/or family.
	See CPT (Evaluation and Management section) for additional coding options.

Available Medical Diagnosis Code(s) - ICD-9-CM **(International Classification of Diseases-9th Revision-Clinical Modification)**	
	See ICD-9-CM Section 520 - 529 (Diseases of Oral Cavity, Salivary Glands, and Jaws) for possible diagnosis codes.

Dental Procedure Code
(Code on Dental Procedures and Nomenclature)
D0210 intraoral – complete series (including bitewings)

Available Medical Procedure Code(s) – CPT
(Current Procedure Terminology)
70320 Radiologic examination, teeth; complete, full mouth

Available Medical Diagnosis Code(s) - ICD-9-CM
(International Classification of Diseases-9th Revision-Clinical Modification)
See ICD-9-CM Section 520 - 529 (Diseases of Oral Cavity, Salivary Glands, and Jaws) for possible diagnosis codes.

. . .

Dental Procedure Code
(Code on Dental Procedures and Nomenclature)
D0220 intraoral – periapical first film

Available Medical Procedure Code(s) – CPT
(Current Procedure Terminology)
70300 Radiologic examination, teeth; single view

Available Medical Diagnosis Code(s) - ICD-9-CM
(International Classification of Diseases-9th Revision-Clinical Modification)
See ICD-9-CM Section 520 - 529 (Diseases of Oral Cavity, Salivary Glands, and Jaws) for possible diagnosis codes.

Dental Procedure Code
(Code on Dental Procedures and Nomenclature)

D0230	intraoral – periapical each additional film

Available Medical Procedure Code(s) – CPT
(Current Procedure Terminology)

70310	Radiologic examination, teeth; partial examination, less than full mouth

Available Medical Diagnosis Code(s) - ICD-9-CM
(International Classification of Diseases-9th Revision-Clinical Modification)

	See ICD-9-CM Section 520 - 529 (Diseases of Oral Cavity, Salivary Glands, and Jaws) for possible diagnosis codes.

. . .

Dental Procedure Code
(Code on Dental Procedures and Nomenclature)

D0320	temporomandibular joint arthrogram, including injection

Available Medical Procedure Code(s) – CPT
(Current Procedure Terminology)

70332	Temporomandibular joint arthrography, radiological supervision and interpretation
21116	Injection procedure for temporomandibular joint arthrography

Available Medical Diagnosis Code(s) - ICD-9-CM
(International Classification of Diseases-9th Revision-Clinical Modification)

524.60	Unspecified temporomandibular joint disorders
	See ICD-9-CM Section 520 - 529 (Diseases of Oral Cavity, Salivary Glands, and Jaws) for additional possible diagnosis codes.

Dental Procedure Code *(Code on Dental Procedures and Nomenclature)*
D0321   other temporomandibular joint films, by report

Available Medical Procedure Code(s) – CPT (Current Procedure Terminology)	
70328	Radiologic examination, temporomandibular joint, open and closed mouth; unilateral
70330	Radiologic examination, temporomandibular joint, open and closed mouth; bilateral

Available Medical Diagnosis Code(s) - ICD-9-CM (International Classification of Diseases-9th Revision-Clinical Modification)	
524.60	Unspecified temporomandibular joint disorders
	See ICD-9-CM Section 520 - 529 (Diseases of Oral Cavity, Salivary Glands, and Jaws) for possible additional diagnosis codes.

. . .

Dental Procedure Code *(Code on Dental Procedures and Nomenclature)*
D0330   panoramic film

Available Medical Procedure Code(s) – CPT (Current Procedure Terminology)	
70355	Orthopantogram

Available Medical Diagnosis Code(s) - ICD-9-CM (International Classification of Diseases-9th Revi sion-Clinical Modification)	
	See ICD-9-CM Section 520 - 529 (Diseases of Oral Cavity, Salivary Glands, and Jaws) for possible diagnosis codes.

Dental Procedure Code *(Code on Dental Procedures and Nomenclature)*	
D0340	cephalometric film
Available Medical Procedure Code(s) – CPT (Current Procedure Terminology)	
70350	Cephalogram, orthodontic
Available Medical Diagnosis Code(s) - ICD-9-CM (International Classification of Diseases-9th Revision-Clinical Modification)	
524.4	Unspecified malocclusion
	See ICD-9-CM Section 520 - 529 (Diseases of Oral Cavity, Salivary Glands, and Jaws) for possible diagnosis codes.

II. Endodontics

Dental Procedure Code *(Code on Dental Procedures and Nomenclature)*	
D3410	apicoectomy/periradicular surgery – anterior
D3421	apicoectomy/periradicular surgery – bicuspid (first root)
D3425	apicoectomy/periradicular surgery – molar (first root)
D3426	apicoectomy/periradicular surgery – (each additional root)
Available Medical Procedure Code(s) – CPT (Current Procedure Terminology)	
41899	Unlisted procedure, dentoalveolar structures (Note: Include narrative that explains circumstances and describes procedure.)
Available Medical Diagnosis Code(s) - ICD-9-CM (International Classification of Diseases-9th Revision-Clinical Modification)	
522.4	Acute apical periodontitis of pulpal origin
522.8	Radicular cyst
522.9	Other and unspecified diseases of pulp and periapical tissues
	See ICD-9-CM Section 520 - 529 (Diseases of Oral Cavity, Salivary Glands, and Jaws) for possible additional diagnosis codes.

Dental Procedure Code *(Code on Dental Procedures and Nomenclature)*	
D3430	retrograde filling – per root
Available Medical Procedure Code(s) – CPT **(Current Procedure Terminology)**	
41899	Unlisted procedure, dentoalveolar structures (Note: Include narrative that explains circumstances and describes procedure.)
Available Medical Diagnosis Code(s) - ICD-9-CM **(International Classification of Diseases-9th Revision-Clinical Modification)**	
522.4	Acute apical periodontitis of pulpal origin
522.8	Radicular cyst
522.9	Other and unspecified diseases of pulp and periapical tissues
	See ICD-9-CM Section 520 - 529 (Diseases of Oral Cavity, Salivary Glands, and Jaws) for possible additional diagnosis codes.

. . .

Dental Procedure Code *(Code on Dental Procedures and Nomenclature)*	
D3450	root amputation – per root
Available Medical Procedure Code(s) – CPT **(Current Procedure Terminology)**	
41899	Unlisted procedure, dentoalveolar structures (Note: Include narrative that explains circumstances and describes procedure.)
Available Medical Diagnosis Code(s) - ICD-9-CM **(International Classification of Diseases-9th Revision-Clinical Modification)**	
522.4	Acute apical periodontitis of pulpal origin
522.8	Radicular cyst
522.9	Other and unspecified diseases of pulp and periapical tissues
	See ICD-9-CM Section 520 - 529 (Diseases of Oral Cavity, Salivary Glands, and Jaws) for possible additional diagnosis codes.

Dental Procedure Code (Code on Dental Procedures and Nomenclature)	
D3470	intentional reimplantation (including necessary splinting)
Available Medical Procedure Code(s) – CPT (Current Procedure Terminology)	
41899	Unlisted procedure, dentoalveolar structures (Note: Include narrative that explains circumstances and describes procedure.)
Available Medical Diagnosis Code(s) - ICD-9-CM (International Classification of Diseases-9th Revision-Clinical Modification)	
522.4	Acute apical periodontitis of pulpal origin
522.8	Radicular cyst
522.9	Other and unspecified diseases of pulp and periapical tissues
	See ICD-9-CM Section 520 - 529 (Diseases of Oral Cavity, Salivary Glands, and Jaws) for possible additional diagnosis codes.

III. Periodontics

	Dental Procedure Code *(Code on Dental Procedures and Nomenclature)*
D4210	gingivectomy or gingivoplasty – four or more contiguous teeth or tooth bounded spaces per quadrant
D4211	gingivectomy or gingivoplasty – one to three contiguous teeth or tooth bounded spaces per quadrant
	Available Medical Procedure Code(s) – CPT **(Current Procedure Terminology)**
41820	Gingivectomy, excision gingiva, each quadrant
41872	Gingivoplasty, each quadrant
	Available Medical Diagnosis Code(s) - ICD-9-CM **(International Classification of Diseases-9th Revision-Clinical Modification)**
523.00	Acute gingivitis, plaque induced
523.10	Chronic gingivitis, plaque induced
523.33	Aggressive periodontitis
523.41	Chronic periodontitis, localized
	See ICD-9-CM Section 520 - 529 (Diseases of Oral Cavity, Salivary Glands, and Jaws) for possible additional diagnosis codes.

Dental Procedure Code *(Code on Dental Procedures and Nomenclature)*	
D4230	anatomical crown exposure – four or more contiguous teeth per quadrant
D4231	anatomical crown exposure – one to three teeth per quadrant
Available Medical Procedure Code(s) – CPT **(Current Procedure Terminology)**	
41899	Unlisted procedure, dentoalveolar structure (Note: Include narrative that explains circumstances and describes procedure.)
Available Medical Diagnosis Code(s) - ICD-9-CM **(International Classification of Diseases-9th Revision-Clinical Modification)**	
524.81	Anterior soft tissue impingement
524.82	Posterior soft tissue impingement
523.8	Other specified periodontal diseases
	See ICD-9-CM Section 520 - 529 (Diseases of Oral Cavity, Salivary Glands, and Jaws) for possible additional diagnosis codes.

· · ·

Dental Procedure Code *(Code on Dental Procedures and Nomenclature)*	
D4240	gingival flap procedure, including root planing – four or more contiguous teeth or tooth bounded spaces per quadrant
D4241	gingival flap procedure, including root planing – one to three contiguous teeth or tooth bounded spaces per quadrant
Available Medical Procedure Code(s) – CPT **(Current Procedure Terminology)**	
41899	Unlisted procedure, dentoalveolar structure (Note: Include narrative that explains circumstances and describes procedure.)
	See current CPT manual for possible additional procedure codes.
Available Medical Diagnosis Code(s) - ICD-9-CM **(International Classification of Diseases-9th Revision-Clinical Modification)**	
523.33	Aggressive periodontitis
523.42	Chronic periodontitis, generalized
523.9	Unspecified gingival and periodontal disease
	See ICD-9-CM Section 520 - 529 (Diseases of Oral Cavity, Salivary Glands, and Jaws) for possible additional diagnosis codes.

Dental Procedure Code
(Code on Dental Procedures and Nomenclature)

D4245	apically positioned flap

Available Medical Procedure Code(s) – CPT
(Current Procedure Terminology)

41899	Unlisted procedure, dentoalveolar structure (Note: Include narrative that explains circumstances and describes procedure.)

Available Medical Diagnosis Code(s) - ICD-9-CM
(International Classification of Diseases-9th Revision-Clinical Modification)

523.21	Gingival recession, moderate
523.10	Chronic gingivitis, plaque induced
523.25	Gingival recession, generalized
523.40	Chronic periodontitis, unspecified
523.9	Unspecified gingival and periodontal disease
	See ICD-9-CM Section 520 - 529 (Diseases of Oral Cavity, Salivary Glands, and Jaws) for possible additional diagnosis codes.

· · ·

Dental Procedure Code
(Code on Dental Procedures and Nomenclature)

D4249	clinical crown lengthening – hard tissue

Available Medical Procedure Code(s) – CPT
(Current Procedure Terminology)

41899	Unlisted procedure, dentoalveolar structures (Note: Include narrative that explains circumstances and describes procedure.)

Available Medical Diagnosis Code(s) - ICD-9-CM
(International Classification of Diseases-9th Revision-Clinical Modification)

521.00	Dental caries, unspecified
873.63	Tooth (broken)
	See ICD-9-CM for possible additional diagnosis codes.

Dental Procedure Code *(Code on Dental Procedures and Nomenclature)*	
D4260	osseous surgery (including flap entry and closure) – four or more contiguous teeth or tooth bounded spaces per quadrant
D4261	osseous surgery (including flap entry and closure) – one to three contiguous teeth or tooth bounded spaces per quadrant
Available Medical Procedure Code(s) – CPT (Current Procedure Terminology)	
41899	Unlisted procedure, dentoalveolar structures (Note: Include narrative that explains circumstances and describes procedure.)
Available Medical Diagnosis Code(s) - ICD-9-CM (International Classification of Diseases-9th Revision-Clinical Modification)	
523.8	Other specified periodontal disease
523.10	Chronic gingivitis, plaque induced
523.42	Chronic periodontitis, generalized
	See ICD-9-CM Section 520 - 529 (Diseases of Oral Cavity, Salivary Glands, and Jaws) for possible additional diagnosis codes.

Dental Procedure Code *(Code on Dental Procedures and Nomenclature)*	
D4266	guided tissue regeneration - resorbable barrier, per site
D4267	guided tissue regeneration - nonresorbable barrier, per site (includes membrane removal)
Available Medical Procedure Code(s) – CPT (Current Procedure Terminology)	
41899	Unlisted procedure, dentoalveolar structures (Note: Include narrative that explains circumstances and describes procedure.)
	See current CPT manual for possible additional procedure codes.
Available Medical Diagnosis Code(s) - ICD-9-CM (International Classification of Diseases-9th Revision-Clinical Modification)	
523.22	Gingival recession, moderate
523.23	Gingival recession, severe
525.23	Severe atrophy of the mandible
525.26	Severe atrophy of the maxilla
	See ICD-9-CM Section 520 - 529 (Diseases of Oral Cavity, Salivary Glands, and Jaws) for possible additional diagnosis codes.

Dental Procedure Code *(Code on Dental Procedures and Nomenclature)*	
D4270	pedicle soft tissue graft
D4271	free soft tissue graft procedure (including donor site surgery)
D4273	subepithelial connective tissue graft procedures, per tooth
D4275	soft tissue allograft
D4276	combined connective tissue and double pedicle graft, per tooth
Available Medical Procedure Code(s) – CPT **(Current Procedure Terminology)**	
41870	Periodontal mucosal grafting
Available Medical Diagnosis Code(s) - ICD-9-CM **(International Classification of Diseases-9th Revision-Clinical Modification)**	
523.22	Gingival recession, moderate
523.23	Gingival recession, severe
523.32	Aggressive periodontitis, generalized
523.41	Chronic periodontitis, localized
	See ICD-9-CM Section 520 - 529 (Diseases of Oral Cavity, Salivary Glands, and Jaws) for possible additional diagnosis codes.

IV. Maxillofacial Prosthodontics

Dental Procedure Code *(Code on Dental Procedures and Nomenclature)*	
D5931	obturator prosthesis, surgical
D5932	obturator prosthesis, definitive
D5936	obturator prosthesis, interim
Available Medical Procedure Code(s) – CPT (Current Procedure Terminology)	
21076	Impression and custom preparation; surgical obturator prosthesis
21079	Impression and custom preparation; interim obturator prosthesis
21080	Impression and custom preparation; definitive obturator prosthesis
	CPT codes 21076, 21079 and 21080 should only be used when the practitioner actually designs and prepares the prosthesis (i.e., not prepared by an outside laboratory)
Available Medical Diagnosis Code(s) - ICD-9-CM (International Classification of Diseases-9th Revision-Clinical Modification)	
749.00	Cleft palate, unspecified
145.2	Neoplasm, malignant, hard palate
	See ICD-9-CM Section 520 - 529 (Diseases of Oral Cavity, Salivary Glands, and Jaws) for possible additional diagnosis codes.

Sleep Apnea Device

Dental Procedure Code *(Code on Dental Procedures and Nomenclature)*	
D5999	unspecified maxillofacial prosthesis, by report
Available Medical Procedure Code(s) – CPT **(Current Procedure Terminology)**	
21089	Unlisted maxillofacial prosthetic procedure CPT code 21089 should only be used when the practitioner actually designs and prepares the prosthesis (i.e., not prepared by an outside laboratory) (Note: Include narrative that explains circumstances and describes procedure.)
Available Medical Procedure Code(s) – HCPCS *(Healthcare Common Procedure Coding System)*	
E0485	*oral device/appliance used to reduce upper airway collapsibility, adjustable or non-adjustable, prefabricated, includes fitting and adjustment*
E0486	*oral device/appliance used to reduce upper airway collapsibility, adjustable or non-adjustable, custom fabricated, includes fitting and adjustment*
Available Medical Diagnosis Code(s) - ICD-9-CM **(International Classification of Diseases-9th Revision-Clinical Modification)**	
327.23	Obstructive sleep apnea (adult) (pediatric)
327.29	Other organic sleep apnea
	See ICD-9-CM Section 327.20 – 327.29 (Nervous system and sense organs) for possible additional diagnosis codes.

V. Implant Services

Dental Procedure Code *(Code on Dental Procedures and Nomenclature)*	
D6010	surgical placement of implant body: endosteal implant
D6012	surgical placement of interim implant body for transitional prosthesis: endosteal implant
D6040	surgical placement: eposteal implant
D6050	surgical placement: transosteal implant
Available Medical Procedure Code(s) – CPT **(Current Procedure Terminology)**	
21248	Reconstruction of mandible or maxilla, endosteal implant (e.g., blade, cylinder); partial
21249	Reconstruction of mandible or maxilla, endosteal implant (e.g., blade, cylinder); complete
	See current CPT manual for possible additional procedure codes.
Available Medical Diagnosis Code(s) - ICD-9-CM **(International Classification of Diseases-9th Revision-Clinical Modification)**	
525.51	Partial edentulism, class I
525.41	Complete edentulism, class I
525.11	Loss of teeth due to trauma
525.12	Loss of teeth due to periodontal disease
	See ICD-9-CM Section 520 - 529 (Diseases of Oral Cavity, Salivary Glands, and Jaws) for possible additional diagnosis codes.

Dental Procedure Code *(Code on Dental Procedures and Nomenclature)*	
D6100	implant removal, by report
Available Medical Procedure Code(s) – CPT (Current Procedure Terminology)	
20670	Removal of implant; superficial (e.g., buried wire, pin or rod) (separate procedure)
20680	Removal of implant; deep (e.g., buried wire, pin, screw, metal band, nail, rod or plate)
	See current CPT manual for possible additional procedure codes.
Available Medical Diagnosis Code(s) - ICD-9-CM (International Classification of Diseases-9th Revision-Clinical Modification)	
996.60	Infection and inflammatory reaction due to internal prosthetic device, implant, and graft (Due to unspecified device, implant, and graft)
996.70	Other complications of internal (biological) (synthetic) prosthetic device, implant, and graft (Due to unspecified device, implant, and graft)
	See ICD-9-CM Section 520 - 529 (Diseases of Oral Cavity, Salivary Glands, and Jaws) for possible additional diagnosis codes.

Dental Procedure Code *(Code on Dental Procedures and Nomenclature)*	
D6190	radiographic/surgical implant index, by report
Available Medical Procedure Code(s) – CPT **(Current Procedure Terminology)**	
41899	Unlisted procedure, dentoalveolar structures (Note: Include narrative that explains circumstances and describes procedure.)
Available Medical Diagnosis Code(s) - ICD-9-CM **(International Classification of Diseases-9th Revision-Clinical Modification)**	
525.10	Acquired absence of teeth, unspecified
525.20	Unspecified atrophy of edentulous alveolar ridge
	See ICD-9-CM Section 520 - 529 (Diseases of Oral Cavity, Salivary Glands, and Jaws) for possible additional diagnosis codes.

VI. Oral and Maxillofacial Surgery

Dental Procedure Code (Code on Dental Procedures and Nomenclature)	
D7210	surgical removal of erupted tooth requiring removal of bone and/or sectioning of tooth, and including elevation of mucoperiosteal flap if indicated
D7220	removal of impacted tooth – soft tissue
D7230	removal of impacted tooth – partial bony
D7240	removal of impacted tooth – complete bony
D7241	removal of impacted tooth – completely bony, with unusual surgical complications
Available Medical Procedure Code(s) – CPT (Current Procedure Terminology)	
41899	Unlisted procedure, dentoalveolar structures (Note: Include narrative that explains circumstances and describes procedure.)
Available Medical Diagnosis Code(s) - ICD-9-CM (International Classification of Diseases-9th Revision-Clinical Modification)	
520.1	Supernumerary teeth
520.6	Disturbances of tooth eruption (includes impacted teeth)
521.00	Dental caries, unspecified
	See ICD-9-CM Section 520 - 529 (Diseases of Oral Cavity, Salivary Glands, and Jaws) for possible additional diagnosis codes.

Dental Procedure Code
(Code on Dental Procedures and Nomenclature)

D7250	surgical removal of residual tooth roots (cutting procedure)

Available Medical Procedure Code(s) – CPT
(Current Procedure Terminology)

41899	Unlisted procedure, dentoalveolar structures (Note: Include narrative that explains circumstances and describes procedure.)

Available Medical Diagnosis Code(s) - ICD-9-CM
(International Classification of Diseases-9th Revision-Clinical Modification)

525.3	Retained dental root
	See ICD-9-CM Section 520 - 529 (Diseases of Oral Cavity, Salivary Glands, and Jaws) for possible additional diagnosis codes.

. . .

Dental Procedure Code
(Code on Dental Procedures and Nomenclature)

D7260	oroantral fistula closure

Available Medical Procedure Code(s) – CPT
(Current Procedure Terminology)

30580	Repair fistula; oromaxillary (combine with 31030 if antrotomy is included)
	See current CPT manual for possible additional procedure codes.

Available Medical Diagnosis Code(s) - ICD-9-CM
(International Classification of Diseases-9th Revision-Clinical Modification)

522.7	Abscess, periapical w/sinus
524.3	Anomaly, tooth position, fully erupt teeth
	See ICD-9-CM Section 520 - 529 (Diseases of Oral Cavity, Salivary Glands, and Jaws) for possible additional diagnosis codes.

Dental Procedure Code
(Code on Dental Procedures and Nomenclature)
D7270	tooth reimplantation and/or stabilization of accidentally evulsed or displaced tooth

Available Medical Procedure Code(s) – CPT
(Current Procedure Terminology)
41899	Unlisted procedure, dentoalveolar structures (Note: Include narrative that explains circumstances and describes procedure.)
	See current CPT manual for possible additional procedure codes.

Available Medical Diagnosis Code(s) - ICD-9-CM
(International Classification of Diseases-9th Revision-Clinical Modification)
524.30	Unspecified anomaly of tooth position (includes displacement of teeth)
	See ICD-9-CM for possible additional diagnosis codes.

· · ·

Dental Procedure Code
(Code on Dental Procedures and Nomenclature)
D7285	biopsy of oral tissue - hard (bone, tooth)

Available Medical Procedure Code(s) – CPT
(Current Procedure Terminology)
20240	Biopsy, bone, open; superficial (eg, ilium, sternum, spinous process, ribs, trochanter of femur)
20245	Biopsy, bone, open; deep (eg, humerus, ischium, femur)
	See current CPT manual for possible additional procedure codes.

Available Medical Diagnosis Code(s) - ICD-9-CM
(International Classification of Diseases-9th Revision-Clinical Modification)
170.0	Neoplasm, malignant, skull/face bones
170.1	Neoplasm, malignant, mandible
213.0	Neoplasm, benign, bone skull/face
213.1	Neoplasm, benign, lower jaw
	See ICD-9-CM for possible additional diagnosis codes.

Dental Procedure Code *(Code on Dental Procedures and Nomenclature)*

D7286	biopsy of oral tissue - soft

Available Medical Procedure Code(s) – CPT **(Current Procedure Terminology)**	
11100	Biopsy of skin, subcutaneous tissue and/or mucous membrane (including simple closure), unless otherwise listed; single lesion
11101	Biopsy of skin, subcutaneous tissue and/or mucous membrane (including simple closure), unless otherwise listed; each separate/ additional lesion (List separately in addition to code for primary procedure)
40490	Biopsy of lip
40808	Biopsy, vestibule of mouth
41100	Biopsy of tongue; anterior two-thirds
41105	Biopsy of tongue; posterior one-third
41108	Biopsy of floor of mouth
42100	Biopsy of palate, uvula
	See current CPT manual for possible additional procedure codes.

Available Medical Diagnosis Code(s) - ICD-9-CM **(International Classification of Diseases-9th Revision-Clinical Modification)**	
528.6	Leukoplakia, oral mucosa including tongue
701.5	Abnormal granulation tissue NEC
	See ICD-9-CM for possible additional diagnosis codes.

Dental Procedure Code (Code on Dental Procedures and Nomenclature)	
D7288	brush biopsy – transepithelial sample collection
Available Medical Procedure Code(s) – CPT **(Current Procedure Terminology)**	
40799	Unlisted procedure, lips (Note: Include narrative that explains circumstances and describes procedure.)
40899	Unlisted procedure, vestibule of mouth (Note: Include narrative that explains circumstances and describes procedure.)
41599	Unlisted procedure, tongue, floor of mouth (Note: Include narrative that explains circumstances and describes procedure.)
	See current CPT manual for possible additional procedure codes.
Available Medical Diagnosis Code(s) - ICD-9-CM **(International Classification of Diseases-9th Revision-Clinical Modification)**	
528.6	Leukoplakia, oral mucosa including tongue
701.5	Abnormal granulation tissue NEC
	See ICD-9-CM for possible additional diagnosis codes.

Dental Procedure Code *(Code on Dental Procedures and Nomenclature)*

D7310	alveoloplasty in conjunction with extractions – four or more teeth or tooth spaces, per quadrant
D7311	alveoloplasty in conjunction with extractions – one to three teeth or tooth spaces, per quadrant
D7320	alveoloplasty not in conjunction with extractions –four or more teeth or tooth spaces, per quadrant
D7321	alveoloplasty not in conjunction with extractions one to three teeth or tooth spaces, per quadrant

Available Medical Procedure Code(s) – CPT **(Current Procedure Terminology)**

41874	Alveoloplasty, each quadrant (specify)

Available Medical Diagnosis Code(s) - ICD-9-CM **(International Classification of Diseases-9th Revision-Clinical Modification)**

524.70	Unspecified alveolar anomaly
525.40	Complete edentulism, unspecified
525.50	Partial edentulism, unspecified
	See ICD-9-CM Section 520 - 529 (Diseases of Oral Cavity, Salivary Glands, and Jaws) for possible additional diagnosis codes.

Dental Procedure Code *(Code on Dental Procedures and Nomenclature)*	
D7340	vestibuloplasty - ridge extension (secondary epithelialization)
Available Medical Procedure Code(s) – CPT **(Current Procedure Terminology)**	
40840	Vestibuloplasty; anterior
40842	Vestibuloplasty; posterior, unilateral
40843	Vestibuloplasty; posterior, bilateral
40844	Vestibuloplasty; entire arch
Available Medical Diagnosis Code(s) - ICD-9-CM **(International Classification of Diseases-9th Revision-Clinical Modification)**	
145.1	Neoplasm, malignant, mouth vestibule
525.20	Unspecified atrophy of edentulous alveolar ridge
	See ICD-9-CM for possible additional diagnosis codes.

. . .

Dental Procedure Code *(Code on Dental Procedures and Nomenclature)*	
D7350	vestibuloplasty - ridge extension (including soft tissue grafts, muscle reattachment, revision of soft tissue attachment and management of hypertrophied and hyperplastic tissue)
Available Medical Procedure Code(s) – CPT **(Current Procedure Terminology)**	
40845	Vestibuloplasty; complex (including ridge extension, muscle repositioning)
Available Medical Diagnosis Code(s) - ICD-9-CM **(International Classification of Diseases-9th Revision-Clinical Modification)**	
145.1	Neoplasm, malignant, mouth vestibule
525.20	Unspecified atrophy of edentulous alveolar ridge
	See ICD-9-CM for possible additional diagnosis codes.

Dental Procedure Code *(Code on Dental Procedures and Nomenclature)*	
D7410	excision of benign lesion up to 1.25 cm
D7411	excision of benign lesion greater than 1.25 cm
D7412	excision of benign lesion, complicated
Available Medical Procedure Code(s) – CPT **(Current Procedure Terminology)**	
40810	Excision of lesion of mucosa and submucosa, vestibule of mouth; without repair
40812	Excision of lesion of mucosa and submucosa, vestibule of mouth; with simple repair
40814	Excision of lesion of mucosa and submucosa, vestibular of mouth; with complex repair
41110	Excision of lesion of tongue without closure
41112	Excision of lesion of tongue with closure; anterior two-thirds
41113	Excision of lesion of tongue with closure; posterior one-third
41114	Excision of lesion of tongue with closure; with local tongue flap (List 41114 in addition to code 41112 or 41113)
41116	Excision, lesion of floor of mouth
11441	Excision, other benign lesion including margins, except skin tag (unless listed elsewhere), face, ears, eyelids, nose , lips, mucous membrane; excised diameter 0.6 to 1.0 cm
	See current CPT manual for possible additional procedure codes.
Available Medical Diagnosis Code(s) - ICD-9-CM **(International Classification of Diseases-9th Revision-Clinical Modification)**	
210.4	Benign neoplasm of other and unspecified parts of the mouth
215.0	Other benign neoplasm of connective and other soft tissue of head, face, neck
528.6	Leukoplakia, oral mucosa including tongue
	See ICD-9-CM for possible additional diagnosis codes.

Dental Procedure Code (Code on Dental Procedures and Nomenclature)	
D7413	excision of malignant lesion up to 1.25 cm
D7414	excision of malignant lesion greater than 1.25 cm
D7415	excision of malignant lesion, complicated
Available Medical Procedure Code(s) – CPT (Current Procedure Terminology)	
40810	Excision of lesion of mucosa and submucosa, vestibule of mouth; without repair
40812	Excision of lesion of mucosa and submucosa, vestibule of mouth; with simple repair
40814	Excision of lesion of mucosa and submucosa, vestibular of mouth; with complex repair
41110	Excision of lesion of tongue without closure
41112	Excision of lesion of tongue with closure; anterior two-thirds
41113	Excision of lesion of tongue with closure; posterior one-third
41114	Excision of lesion of tongue with closure; with local tongue flap (List 41114 in addition to code 41112 or 41113)
41116	Excision, lesion of floor of mouth
11641	Excision, malignant lesion including margins, face, ears, eyelids, nose, lips; excised diameter 0.6 to 1.0cm
	See current CPT manual for possible additional procedure codes.
Available Medical Diagnosis Code(s) - ICD-9-CM (International Classification of Diseases-9th Revision-Clinical Modification)	
144.1	Malignant neoplasm of lateral portion of floor of mouth
141.3	Malignant neoplasm of ventral surface of tongue
172.0	Melanoma, malignant, lip
	See ICD-9-CM for possible additional diagnosis codes.

	Dental Procedure Code *(Code on Dental Procedures and Nomenclature)*
D7440	excision of malignant tumor - lesion diameter up to 1.25 cm
D7441	excision of malignant tumor - lesion diameter greater than 1.25 cm
	Available Medical Procedure Code(s) – CPT **(Current Procedure Terminology)**
21044	Excision of malignant tumor of mandible;
21034	Excision of malignant tumor of maxilla or zygoma
41825	Excision of lesion or tumor (except listed above), dentoalveolar structures; without repair
41826	Excision of lesion or tumor (except listed above), dentoalveolar structures; with simple repair
41827	Excision of lesion or tumor (except listed above), dentoalveolar structures; with complex repair
	See current CPT manual for possible additional procedure codes.
	Available Medical Diagnosis Code(s) - ICD-9-CM **(International Classification of Diseases-9th Revision-Clinical Modification)**
170.1	Neoplasm, malignant, mandible
	See ICD-9-CM for possible additional diagnosis codes.

Dental Procedure Code
(Code on Dental Procedures and Nomenclature)
D7465   destruction of lesion(s) by physical or chemical method, by report

Available Medical Procedure Code(s) – CPT
(Current Procedure Terminology)
40820   Destruction of lesion or scar of vestibule of mouth by physical methods (eg, laser, thermal, cryo, chemical)
17000   Destruction (eg, laser surgery, electrosurgery, cryosurgery, chemosurgery, surgical curettement), premalignant lesions (eg, actinic keratoses); first lesion
See also codes 17001-17004 and 17280-17286 in the Integumentary Section of the current CPT manual.

Available Medical Diagnosis Code(s) - ICD-9-CM
(International Classification of Diseases-9th Revision-Clinical Modification)
216.0   Neoplasm, benign, skin, lip
413.1   Malignant neoplasm of lower gum
See ICD-9-CM for possible additional diagnosis codes.

· · ·

Dental Procedure Code
(Code on Dental Procedures and Nomenclature)
D7471   removal of lateral exostosis (maxilla or mandible)
D7472   removal of torus palatinus
D7473   removal of torus mandibularis

Available Medical Procedure Code(s) – CPT
(Current Procedure Terminology)
21031   Excision of torus mandibularis
21032   Excision of maxillary torus palatinus

Available Medical Diagnosis Code(s) - ICD-9-CM
(International Classification of Diseases-9th Revision-Clinical Modification)
526.81   Exostosis, jaw

Dental Procedure Code
(*Code on Dental Procedures and Nomenclature*)

D7485	surgical reduction of osseous tuberosity

Available Medical Procedure Code(s) – CPT
(Current Procedure Terminology)

41823	Excision of osseous tuberosities, dentoalveolar structures

Available Medical Diagnosis Code(s) - ICD-9-CM
(International Classification of Diseases-9th Revision-Clinical Modification)

526.81	Exostosis, jaw

. . .

Dental Procedure Code
(*Code on Dental Procedures and Nomenclature*)

D7490	radical resection of maxilla or mandible

Available Medical Procedure Code(s) – CPT
(Current Procedure Terminology)

21045	Excision of malignant tumor of mandible; radical resection

Available Medical Diagnosis Code(s) - ICD-9-CM
(International Classification of Diseases-9th Revision-Clinical Modification)

179.1	Malignant neoplasm, mandible
	See ICD-9-CM for possible additional diagnosis codes.

Dental Procedure Code	
(Code on Dental Procedures and Nomenclature)	
D7510	incision and drainage of abscess - intraoral soft tissue
D7511	incision and drainage of abscess – intraoral soft tissue - complicated (includes drainage of multiple fascial spaces)
Available Medical Procedure Code(s) – CPT **(Current Procedure Terminology)**	
20000	Incision of soft tissue abscess (e.g., secondary to osteomyelitis): superficial
41000	Intraoral incision and drainage of abscess, cyst, or hematoma of tongue or floor of mouth; lingual
41005	Intraoral incision and drainage of abscess, cyst, or hematoma of tongue or floor of mouth; sublingual, superficial
41015	Extraoral incision and drainage of abscess, cyst, or hematoma of tongue or floor of mouth; sublingual
41017	Extraoral incision and drainage of abscess, cyst, or hematoma of floor of mouth; submandibular
10060	Incision and drainage of abscess (eg, carbuncle, suppurative hidradenitis, cutaneous or subcutaneous abscess, cyst, furuncle, or paronychia); simple or single
	See CPT manual for additional procedure code possibilities, especially the range 41000-41009 for intraoral procedures and 41015-41018 for extraoral procedures.
Available Medical Diagnosis Code(s) - ICD-9-CM **(International Classification of Diseases-9th Revision-Clinical Modification)**	
522.5	Periapical abscess without sinus
682.0	Cellulitis and abscess of face
	See ICD-9-CM for possible additional diagnosis codes.

Dental Procedure Code *(Code on Dental Procedures and Nomenclature)*	
D7520	incision and drainage of abscess – extraoral soft tissue
D7521	incision and drainage of abscess – extraoral soft tissue – complicated (includes drainage of multiple fascial spaces)
Available Medical Procedure Code(s) – CPT **(Current Procedure Terminology)**	
10060	Incision and drainage of abscess (eg, carbuncle, suppurative hidradenitis, and other cutaneous or subcutaneous abscess, cyst, furuncle, or paronychia); simple or single
10061	Incision and drainage of abscess (eg, carbuncle, suppurative hidradenitis, and other cutaneous or subcutaneous abscess, cyst, furuncle, or paronychia); complicated or multiple
41015	Extraoral incision and drainage of abscess, cyst, or hematoma of floor of mouth; sublingual
	See CPT manual for additional procedure code possibilities, especially the range 41016-41018 for additional extraoral procedures.
Available Medical Diagnosis Code(s) - ICD-9-CM **(International Classification of Diseases-9th Revision-Clinical Modification)**	
523.41	Chronic periodontitis
528.3	Cellulitis/abscess, mouth
	See ICD-9-CM Section 520 - 529 (Diseases of Oral Cavity, Salivary Glands, and Jaws) for possible additional diagnosis codes.

Dental Procedure Code
(Code on Dental Procedures and Nomenclature)
D7530 — removal of foreign body from mucosa, skin, or subcutaneous alveolar tissue

Available Medical Procedure Code(s) – CPT (Current Procedure Terminology)	
10120	Incision and removal of foreign body, subcutaneous tissues; simple
10121	Incision and removal of foreign body, subcutaneous tissues; complicated
40804	Removal of embedded foreign body, vestibule of mouth; simple
40805	Removal of embedded foreign body, vestibule of mouth; complicated
41805	Removal of embedded foreign body from dentoalveolar structures; soft tissues
	See current CPT manual for possible additional procedure codes.

Available Medical Diagnosis Code(s) - ICD-9-CM (International Classification of Diseases-9th Revision-Clinical Modification)	
935.0	Foreign body in mouth
	See ICD-9-CM for possible additional diagnosis codes.

. . .

Dental Procedure Code
(Code on Dental Procedures and Nomenclature)
D7540 — removal of reaction producing foreign bodies, musculoskeletal system

Available Medical Procedure Code(s) – CPT (Current Procedure Terminology)	
20520	Removal of foreign body in muscle or tendon sheath; simple
20525	Removal of foreign body in muscle or tendon sheath; deep or complicated
41806	Removal of embedded foreign body from dentoalveolar structures; bone
	See current CPT manual for possible additional procedure codes.

Available Medical Diagnosis Code(s) - ICD-9-CM (International Classification of Diseases-9th Revision-Clinical Modification)	
728.82	Foreign body granuloma muscle
935.0	Foreign body in mouth
	See ICD-9-CM for possible additional diagnosis codes.

Dental Procedure Code
(Code on Dental Procedures and Nomenclature)
D7550 — partial ostectomy/sequestrectomy for removal of non-vital bone
Available Medical Procedure Code(s) – CPT
(Current Procedure Terminology)
41830 — Alveoloectomy, including curettage of osteitis or sequestrectomy
See current CPT manual for possible additional procedure codes.
Available Medical Diagnosis Code(s) - ICD-9-CM
(International Classification of Diseases-9th Revision-Clinical Modification)
523.8 — Disease, periodontal NEC
526.5 — Alveolitis, jaw
See ICD-9-CM for possible additional diagnosis codes.

• • •

Dental Procedure Code
(Code on Dental Procedures and Nomenclature)
D7560 — maxillary sinusotomy for removal of tooth fragment or foreign body
Available Medical Procedure Code(s) – CPT
(Current Procedure Terminology)
31020 — Sinusotomy, maxillary (antrotomy); intranasal
31030 — Sinusotomy, maxillary (antrotomy); radical (Caldwell-Luc) without removal of antrochoanal polyps
See current CPT manual for possible additional procedure codes.
Available Medical Diagnosis Code(s) - ICD-9-CM
(International Classification of Diseases-9th Revision-Clinical Modification)
473.0 — Sinusitis, chromic maxillary
932 — Foreign body, nose
See ICD-9-CM for possible additional diagnosis codes.

Dental Procedure Code *(Code on Dental Procedures and Nomenclature)*	
D7610	maxilla - open reduction (teeth immobilized, if present)
D7630	mandible - open reduction (teeth immobilized, if present)
Available Medical Procedure Code(s) – CPT **(Current Procedure Terminology)**	
21432	Open treatment of craniofacial separation (LeFort III type); with wiring and/or internal fixation
21462	Open treatment of mandibular fracture; with interdental fixation
	See current CPT manual for possible additional procedure codes.
Available Medical Diagnosis Code(s) - ICD-9-CM **(International Classification of Diseases-9th Revision-Clinical Modification)**	
524.75	Displacement, vertical, alveolus and teeth
524.76	Deviation, occlusal plane
	See ICD-9-CM for possible additional diagnosis codes.

· · ·

Dental Procedure Code *(Code on Dental Procedures and Nomenclature)*	
D7620	maxilla - closed reduction (teeth immobilized, if present)
D7640	mandible - closed reduction (teeth immobilized, if present)
Available Medical Procedure Code(s) - CPT **(Current Procedure Terminology)**	
21440	Closed treatment of mandibular or maxillary alveolar ridge fracture (separate procedure)
21450	Closed treatment of mandibular fracture; without manipulation
21451	Closed treatment of mandibular fracture; with manipulation
	See current CPT manual for possible additional procedure codes.
Available Medical Diagnosis Code(s) - ICD-9-CM **(International Classification of Diseases-9th Revision-Clinical Modification)**	
524.75	Displacement, vertical, alveolus and teeth
802.38	Fracture, symphysis, mandible body open
	See ICD-9-CM for possible additional diagnosis codes.

Dental Procedure Code *(Code on Dental Procedures and Nomenclature)*	
D7650	malar and/or zygomatic arch - open reduction
D7660	malar and/or zygomatic arch - closed reduction
Available Medical Procedure Code(s) – CPT **(Current Procedure Terminology)**	
21356	Open treatment of depressed zygomatic arch fracture (eg, Gilles approach)
21360	Open treatment of depressed malar fracture, including zygomatic arch and malar tripod
	See current CPT manual for possible additional procedure codes.
Available Medical Diagnosis Code(s) - ICD-9-CM **(International Classification of Diseases-9th Revision-Clinical Modification)**	
802.4	Fracture, malar/maxillary, closed
802.5	Fracture, malar/maxillary, open
	See ICD-9-CM for possible additional diagnosis codes.

. . .

Dental Procedure Code *(Code on Dental Procedures and Nomenclature)*	
D7670	alveolus - closed reduction, may include stabilization of teeth
D7671	alveolus - open reduction, may include stabilization of teeth
Available Medical Procedure Code(s) – CPT **(Current Procedure Terminology)**	
21440	Closed treatment of mandibular or maxillary alveolar ridge fracture (separate procedure)
21445	Open treatment of mandibular or maxillary alveolar ridge fracture (separate procedure)
	See current CPT manual for possible additional procedure codes.
Available Medical Diagnosis Code(s) - ICD-9-CM **(International Classification of Diseases-9th Revision-Clinical Modification)**	
802.27	Fracture, alveolar border, mandible body, closed
802.37	Fracture, alveolar border, mandible body, open
	See ICD-9-CM for possible additional diagnosis codes.

Dental Procedure Code	
(Code on Dental Procedures and Nomenclature)	
D7680	facial bones - complicated reduction with fixation and multiple surgical approaches
Available Medical Procedure Code(s) – CPT	
(Current Procedure Terminology)	
	See CPT manual for procedure code possibilities (eg, codes 21310-21497).
Available Medical Diagnosis Code(s) - ICD-9-CM	
(International Classification of Diseases-9th Revision-Clinical Modification)	
820.0	Fracture, nasal bone, closed
802.5	Fracture, malar/maxillary, open
	See ICD-9-CM for possible additional diagnosis codes.

. . .

Dental Procedure Code	
(Code on Dental Procedures and Nomenclature)	
D7710	maxilla - open reduction
D7730	mandible - open reduction
Available Medical Procedure Code(s) – CPT	
(Current Procedure Terminology)	
21422	Open treatment of palatal or maxillary fracture (LeFort I type);
21465	Open treatment of mandibular condylar fracture
21461	Open treatment of mandibular fracture; without interdental fixation
	See current CPT manual for possible additional procedure codes.
Available Medical Diagnosis Code(s) - ICD-9-CM	
(International Classification of Diseases-9th Revision-Clinical Modification)	
524.75	Displacement, vertical, alveolus and teeth
802.32	Mandibular subcondylar process fracture, open
	See ICD-9-CM for possible additional diagnosis codes.

Dental Procedure Code *(Code on Dental Procedures and Nomenclature)*	
D7720	maxilla - closed reduction
D7740	mandible - closed reduction
Available Medical Procedure Code(s) – CPT **(Current Procedure Terminology)**	
21421	Closed treatment of palatal or maxillary fracture (LeFort I type), with interdental wire fixation or fixation of denture or splint
21450	Closed treatment of mandibular fracture; without manipulation
	See current CPT manual for possible additional procedure codes.
Available Medical Diagnosis Code(s) - ICD-9-CM **(International Classification of Diseases-9th Revision-Clinical Modification)**	
524.75	Displacement, vertical, alveolus and teeth
524.76	Deviation, occlusal plane
	See ICD-9-CM for possible additional diagnosis codes.

. . .

Dental Procedure Code *(Code on Dental Procedures and Nomenclature)*	
D7750	malar and/or zygomatic arch - open reduction
D7760	malar and/or zygomatic arch - closed reduction
Available Medical Procedure Code(s) – CPT **(Current Procedure Terminology)**	
21360	Open treatment of depressed malar fracture, including zygomatic arch and malar tripod
	See current CPT manual for possible additional procedure codes.
Available Medical Diagnosis Code(s) - ICD-9-CM **(International Classification of Diseases-9th Revision-Clinical Modification)**	
802.4	Fracture, malar / maxillary, closed
802.5	Fracture, malar / maxillary, open
	See ICD-9-CM for possible additional diagnosis codes.

Dental Procedure Code	
(Code on Dental Procedures and Nomenclature)	
D7770	alveolus - open reduction stabilization of teeth
D7771	alveolus, closed reduction stabilization of teeth
Available Medical Procedure Code(s) – CPT **(Current Procedure Terminology)**	
21440	Closed treatment of mandibular or maxillary alveolar ridge fracture (separate procedure)
21445	Open treatment of mandibular or maxillary alveolar ridge fracture (separate procedure)
Available Medical Diagnosis Code(s) - ICD-9-CM **(International Classification of Diseases-9th Revision-Clinical Modification)**	
802.27	Fracture, alveolar border, mandible body, closed
802.37	Fracture, alveolar border, mandible body, open
	See ICD-9-CM for possible additional diagnosis codes.

• • •

Dental Procedure Code	
(Code on Dental Procedures and Nomenclature)	
D7780	facial bones - complicated reduction with fixation and multiple surgical approaches
Available Medical Procedure Code(s) – CPT **(Current Procedure Terminology)**	
	See CPT manual for procedure code possibilities (eg, codes 21310-21497).
Available Medical Diagnosis Code(s) - ICD-9-CM **(International Classification of Diseases-9th Revision-Clinical Modification)**	
802.1	Fracture, nasal bone, open
802.4	Fracture, malar / maxillary, closed
	See ICD-9-CM for possible additional diagnosis codes.

Dental Procedure Code
(Code on Dental Procedures and Nomenclature)

D7810	open reduction of dislocation
D7820	closed reduction of dislocation

Available Medical Procedure Code(s) – CPT
(Current Procedure Terminology)

21480	Closed treatment of temporomandibular dislocation; initial or subsequent
21485	Closed treatment of temporomandibular dislocation complicated (eg, recurrent requiring intermaxillary fixation or splinting), initial or subsequent
21490	Open treatment of temporomandibular dislocation
	See current CPT manual for possible additional procedure codes.

Available Medical Diagnosis Code(s) - ICD-9-CM
(International Classification of Diseases-9th Revision-Clinical Modification)

524.64	Disorder, TMJ, joint sounds on opening and/or closing the jaw
728.85	Spasm, muscle
830.0	Dislocation closed jaw
	See ICD-9-CM for possible additional diagnosis codes.

. . .

Dental Procedure Code
(Code on Dental Procedures and Nomenclature)

D7830	manipulation under anesthesia

Available Medical Procedure Code(s) – CPT
(Current Procedure Terminology)

21073	Manipulation of temporomandibular joint(s) (TMJ), therapeutic, requiring an anesthesia service (ie, general or monitored anesthesia care)

Available Medical Diagnosis Code(s) - ICD-9-CM
(International Classification of Diseases-9th Revision-Clinical Modification)

830.0	Dislocation closed jaw
	See ICD-9-CM for possible additional diagnosis codes.

Dental Procedure Code
(Code on Dental Procedures and Nomenclature)

D7840	condylectomy

Available Medical Procedure Code(s) – CPT
(Current Procedure Terminology)

21050	Condylectomy, temporomandibular joint (separate procedure)

Available Medical Diagnosis Code(s) - ICD-9-CM
(International Classification of Diseases-9th Revision-Clinical Modification)

170.0	Neoplasm, malignant, skull/face bones
802.31	Fracture, condylar process, mandible, open
	See ICD-9-CM for possible additional diagnosis codes.

. . .

Dental Procedure Code
(Code on Dental Procedures and Nomenclature)

D7850	surgical discectomy, with/without implant

Available Medical Procedure Code(s) – CPT
(Current Procedure Terminology)

21060	Meniscectomy, partial or complete, temporomandibular joint (separate procedure)

Available Medical Diagnosis Code(s) - ICD-9-CM
(International Classification of Diseases-9th Revision-Clinical Modification)

524.69	Other specified temporomandibular joint disorders
905.0	Late effect, skull/face fracture
	See ICD-9-CM for possible additional diagnosis codes.

Dental Procedure Code (Code on Dental Procedures and Nomenclature)	
D7852	disc repair
Available Medical Procedure Code(s) – CPT (Current Procedure Terminology)	
21299	Unlisted craniofacial and maxillofacial procedure (Note: Include narrative that explains circumstances and describes procedure.)
Available Medical Diagnosis Code(s) - ICD-9-CM (International Classification of Diseases-9th Revision-Clinical Modification)	
524.69	Other specified temporomandibular joint disorders
	See ICD-9-CM for possible additional diagnosis codes.

. . .

Dental Procedure Code (Code on Dental Procedures and Nomenclature)	
D7854	synovectomy
Available Medical Procedure Code(s) – CPT (Current Procedure Terminology)	
21299	Unlisted craniofacial and maxillofacial procedure (Note: Include narrative that explains circumstances and describes procedure.)
Available Medical Diagnosis Code(s) - ICD-9-CM (International Classification of Diseases-9th Revision-Clinical Modification)	
524.69	Other specified temporomandibular joint disorders
	See ICD-9-CM for possible additional diagnosis codes.

Dental Procedure Code
(Code on Dental Procedures and Nomenclature)
D7856   myotomy

Available Medical Procedure Code(s) – CPT
(Current Procedure Terminology)
21299   Unlisted craniofacial and maxillofacial procedure (Note: Include narrative that explains circumstances and describes procedure.)

Available Medical Diagnosis Code(s) - ICD-9-CM
(International Classification of Diseases-9th Revision-Clinical Modification)
524.69   Other specified temporomandibular joint disorders
See ICD-9-CM for possible additional diagnosis codes.

• • •

Dental Procedure Code
(Code on Dental Procedures and Nomenclature)
D7858   joint reconstruction

Available Medical Procedure Code(s) – CPT
(Current Procedure Terminology)
21299   Unlisted craniofacial and maxillofacial procedure (Note: Include narrative that explains circumstances and describes procedure.)

Available Medical Diagnosis Code(s) - ICD-9-CM
(International Classification of Diseases-9th Revision-Clinical Modification)
524.69   Other specified temporomandibular joint disorders
See ICD-9-CM for possible additional diagnosis codes.

Dental Procedure Code
(*Code on Dental Procedures and Nomenclature*)

D7860	arthrotomy

Available Medical Procedure Code(s) – CPT
(**Current Procedure Terminology**)

21010	Arthrotomy, temporomandibular joint

Available Medical Diagnosis Code(s) - ICD-9-CM
(**International Classification of Diseases-9th Revision-Clinical Modification**)

524.79	Anomaly, alveolar
524.69	Other specified temporomandibular joint disorders
	See ICD-9-CM for possible additional diagnosis codes.

. . .

Dental Procedure Code
(*Code on Dental Procedures and Nomenclature*)

D7865	arthroplasty

Available Medical Procedure Code(s) – CPT
(**Current Procedure Terminology**)

21240	Arthroplasty, temporomandibular joint, with or without autograft
21242	Arthroplasty, temporomandibular joint, with allograft

Available Medical Diagnosis Code(s) - ICD-9-CM
(**International Classification of Diseases-9th Revision-Clinical Modification**)

170.0	Neoplasm malignant, skull / face bones
714.0	Arthritis, rheumatoid
	See ICD-9-CM for possible additional diagnosis codes.

Dental Procedure Code (Code on Dental Procedures and Nomenclature)	
D7870	arthrocentesis
Available Medical Procedure Code(s) – CPT **(Current Procedure Terminology)**	
20605	Arthrocentesis, aspiration and/or injection; intermediate joint or bursa (eg, temporomandibular, acromioclavicular, wrist, elbow or ankle, olecranon bursa)
Available Medical Diagnosis Code(s) - ICD-9-CM **(International Classification of Diseases-9th Revision-Clinical Modification)**	
524.64	Disorder, TMJ, joint sounds on opening and/or closing the jaw
526.4	Inflammation, jaw
	See ICD-9-CM for possible additional diagnosis codes.

. . .

Dental Procedure Code (Code on Dental Procedures and Nomenclature)	
D7871	non-arthroscopic lysis and lavage
Available Medical Procedure Code(s) – CPT **(Current Procedure Terminology)**	
41899	Unlisted procedure, dentoalveolar structures (Note: Include narrative that explains circumstances and describes procedure.)
Available Medical Diagnosis Code(s) - ICD-9-CM **(International Classification of Diseases-9th Revision-Clinical Modification)**	
524.64	Disorder, TMJ, joint sounds on opening and/or closing the jaw
526.4	Inflammation, jaw
	See ICD-9-CM for possible additional diagnosis codes.

Dental Procedure Code *(Code on Dental Procedures and Nomenclature)*	
D7872	arthroscopy - diagnosis, with or without biopsy
Available Medical Procedure Code(s) – CPT (Current Procedure Terminology)	
29800	Arthroscopy, temporomandibular joint, diagnostic, with or without synovial biopsy (separate procedure)
Available Medical Diagnosis Code(s) - ICD-9-CM (International Classification of Diseases-9th Revision-Clinical Modification)	
714.0	Arthritis, rheumatoid
848.1	Sprain / strain, jaw
	See ICD-9-CM for possible additional diagnosis codes.

. . .

Dental Procedure Code *(Code on Dental Procedures and Nomenclature)*	
D7873	arthroscopy - surgical: lavage and lysis of adhesions
D7874	arthroscopy - surgical: disc repositioning and stabilization
D7875	arthroscopy - surgical: synovectomy
D7876	arthroscopy - surgical: discectomy
D7877	arthroscopy - surgical: debridement
Available Medical Procedure Code(s) – CPT (Current Procedure Terminology)	
29804	Arthroscopy, temporomandibular joint, surgical
	See current CPT manual for possible additional procedure codes.
Available Medical Diagnosis Code(s) - ICD-9-CM (International Classification of Diseases-9th Revision-Clinical Modification)	
524.64	Disorder, TMJ, joint sounds on opening and/or closing the jaw
802.21	Fracture, condylar process, mandible, closed
803.0	Dislocation closed jaw
	See ICD-9-CM for possible additional diagnosis codes.

Dental Procedure Code *(Code on Dental Procedures and Nomenclature)*
D7880 occlusal orthotic device, by report

Available Medical Procedure Code(s) – CPT (Current Procedure Terminology)
41899 Unlisted procedure, dentoalveolar structures (Note: Include narrative that explains circumstances and describes procedure.)

Available Medical Procedure Code(s) – HCPCS *(Healthcare Common Procedure Coding System)*
S8262 Mandibular orthopedic repositioning device, each

Available Medical Diagnosis Code(s) - ICD-9-CM (International Classification of Diseases-9th Revision-Clinical Modification)
524.60 Temporomandibular joint disorders, unspecified
See ICD-9-CM for possible additional diagnosis codes.

. . .

Dental Procedure Code *(Code on Dental Procedures and Nomenclature)*
D7910 suture of recent small wounds up to 5 cm

Available Medical Procedure Code(s) – CPT (Current Procedure Terminology)
12013 Simple repair of superficial wounds of face, ears, eyelids, nose, lips and or mucous membranes; 2.6 cm to 5.0 cm
40830 Closure of laceration, vestibule of mouth; 2.5 cm or less
40831 Closure of laceration, vestibule of mouth; over 2.5cm or complex
41250 Repair of laceration 2.5 cm or less; floor of mouth and/or anterior two-thirds of tongue
41251 Repair of laceration 2.5 cm or less; posterior one-third of tongue
See current CPT manual for possible additional procedure codes.

Available Medical Diagnosis Code(s) - ICD-9-CM (International Classification of Diseases-9th Revision-Clinical Modification)
873.43 Wound open, lip w/o complications
873.64 Wound open, tongue, floor mouth w/o complications
See ICD-9-CM for possible additional diagnosis codes.

Dental Procedure Code (Code on Dental Procedures and Nomenclature)	
D7911	complicated suture – up to 5 cm
Available Medical Procedure Code(s) – CPT (Current Procedure Terminology)	
12052	Layer closure of wounds of face, ears, eyelids, nose, lips and/or mucous membranes; 2.6cm to 5.0 cm
13152	Repair complex, eyelids, nose, ears and/or lips; 1.1 cm to 2.5 cm
	See current CPT manual for possible additional procedure codes.
Available Medical Diagnosis Code(s) - ICD-9-CM (International Classification of Diseases-9th Revision-Clinical Modification)	
873.53	wound open, lip w/complication
873.79	wound open, mouth NEC w/o complications
	See ICD-9-CM for possible additional diagnosis codes.

· · ·

Dental Procedure Code (Code on Dental Procedures and Nomenclature)	
D7912	complicated suture - greater than 5 cm
Available Medical Procedure Code(s) – CPT (Current Procedure Terminology)	
12053	Layer closure of wounds of face, ears, eyelids, nose, lips and/or mucous membranes; 5.1 cm to 7.5 cm
41252	Repair of laceration of tongue, floor of mouth, over 2.6 cm or complex
	See current CPT manual for possible additional procedure codes.
Available Medical Diagnosis Code(s) - ICD-9-CM (International Classification of Diseases-9th Revision-Clinical Modification)	
873.43	Wound open, lip w/o complication
873.69	Wound open, mouth NEC w/o complication
	See ICD-9-CM for possible additional diagnosis codes.

Dental Procedure Code
(Code on Dental Procedures and Nomenclature)

D7920	skin graft (identify defect covered, location and type of graft)

Available Medical Procedure Code(s) – CPT
(Current Procedure Terminology)

	Please reference the range of codes 15002-15260 in the CPT manual for procedure code possibilities.

Available Medical Diagnosis Code(s) - ICD-9-CM
(International Classification of Diseases-9th Revision-Clinical Modification)

528.9	Disease, oral soft tissue NEC
	See ICD-9-CM for possible additional diagnosis codes.

· · ·

Dental Procedure Code
(Code on Dental Procedures and Nomenclature)

D7940	osteoplasty - for orthognathic deformities

Available Medical Procedure Code(s) – CPT
(Current Procedure Terminology)

21299	Unlisted craniofacial or maxillofacial procedure (Note: Include narrative that explains circumstances and describes procedure.)

Available Medical Diagnosis Code(s) - ICD-9-CM
(International Classification of Diseases-9th Revision-Clinical Modification)

524.04	Mandibular hypoplasia
525.23	Severe atrophy mandible
	See ICD-9-CM for possible additional diagnosis codes.

Dental Procedure Code *(Code on Dental Procedures and Nomenclature)*	
D7941	osteotomy - mandibular rami
D7943	osteotomy - mandibular rami with bone graft; includes obtaining the graft
Available Medical Procedure Code(s) – CPT (Current Procedure Terminology)	
21193	Reconstruction of mandibular rami, horizontal, vertical, C or L osteotomy; without bone graft
21194	Reconstruction of mandibular rami, horizontal, vertical, C or L osteotomy; with bone graft (includes obtaining graft)
	See current CPT manual for possible additional procedure codes.
Available Medical Diagnosis Code(s) - ICD-9-CM (International Classification of Diseases-9th Revision-Clinical Modification)	
524.04	Mandibular hypoplasia
524.75	Displacement, vertical, alveolus and teeth
	See ICD-9-CM for possible additional diagnosis codes.

. . .

Dental Procedure Code *(Code on Dental Procedures and Nomenclature)*	
D7944	osteotomy - segmented or subapical
Available Medical Procedure Code(s) – CPT (Current Procedure Terminology)	
21198	Osteotomy, mandible, segmental
21206	Osteotomy, maxilla, segmental (eg, Wassmund or Schuchard)
	See current CPT manual for possible additional procedure codes.
Available Medical Diagnosis Code(s) - ICD-9-CM (International Classification of Diseases-9th Revision-Clinical Modification)	
524.02	Mandibular hyperplasia
749.01	Cleft palate, unilateral complete
	See ICD-9-CM for possible additional diagnosis codes.

Dental Procedure Code *(Code on Dental Procedures and Nomenclature)*	
D7945	osteotomy - body of mandible
Available Medical Procedure Code(s) – CPT (Current Procedure Terminology)	
21198	Osteotomy, mandible, segmental
	See current CPT manual for possible additional procedure codes.
Available Medical Diagnosis Code(s) - ICD-9-CM (International Classification of Diseases-9th Revision-Clinical Modification)	
524.02	Mandibular hyperplasia
754.0	Deformity, skull / face / jaw congenital
	See ICD-9-CM for possible additional diagnosis codes.

Dental Procedure Code
(Code on Dental Procedures and Nomenclature)

D7946	LeFort I (maxilla - total)

Available Medical Procedure Code(s) – CPT
(Current Procedure Terminology)

21141	Reconstruction midface, LeFort I; single piece, segment movement in any direction (eg, for Long Face Syndrome), without bone graft
21142	Reconstruction midface, LeFort I; two pieces, segment movement in any direction, without bone qraft
21143	Reconstruction midface, LeFort I; three or more pieces, segment movement in any direction, without bone graft
21145	Reconstruction midface, LeFort I; single piece, segment movement in any direction, requiring bone grafts (includes obtaining autografts)
21146	Reconstruction midface, LeFort I; two pieces, segment movement in any direction, requiring bone grafts (includes obtaining autografts) (eg, ungrafted unilateral alveolar cleft)
21147	Reconstruction midface, LeFort I; three or more pieces, segment movement in any direction, requiring bone grafts (includes obtaining autografts) (eg, ungrafted bilateral alveolar cleft or multiple osteotomies)
	See current CPT manual for possible additional procedure codes.

Available Medical Diagnosis Code(s) - ICD-9-CM
(International Classification of Diseases-9th Revision-Clinical Modification)

524.03	Maxillary hypoplasia
754.0	Deformity, skull / face / jaw, congenital
	See ICD-9-CM for possible additional diagnosis codes.

Dental Procedure Code *(Code on Dental Procedures and Nomenclature)*	
D7947	LeFort I (maxilla - segmented)
Available Medical Procedure Code(s) – CPT **(Current Procedure Terminology)**	
21299	Unlisted craniofacial and maxillofacial procedure (Note: Include narrative that explains circumstances and describes procedure.)
Available Medical Diagnosis Code(s) - ICD-9-CM **(International Classification of Diseases-9th Revision-Clinical Modification)**	
524.03	Maxillary hypoplasia
524.20	Unspecified anomaly of dental arch relationship
	See ICD-9-CM for possible additional diagnosis codes.

. . .

Dental Procedure Code *(Code on Dental Procedures and Nomenclature)*	
D7948	LeFort II or LeFort III (osteoplasty of facial bones for midface hypoplasia or retrusion)-without bone graft
Available Medical Procedure Code(s) – CPT **(Current Procedure Terminology)**	
21150	Reconstruction midface, LeFort II; anterior intrusion (e.g., Treacher-Collins Syndrome)
	See current CPT manual for possible additional procedure codes.
Available Medical Diagnosis Code(s) - ICD-9-CM **(International Classification of Diseases-9th Revision-Clinical Modification)**	
526.89	Disease, jaw NEC
754.0	Deformity, skull / face / jaw, congenital
	See ICD-9-CM for possible additional diagnosis codes.

Dental Procedure Code *(Code on Dental Procedures and Nomenclature)*	
D7949	LeFort II or LeFort III – with bone graft
Available Medical Procedure Code(s) – CPT **(Current Procedure Terminology)**	
21154	Reconstruction midface, LeFort III (extracranial), any type, requiring bone grafts (includes obtaining autografts); without LeFort I
21151	Reconstruction midface, LeFort II; any direction, requiring bone grafts (includes obtaining autografts)
21159	Reconstruction midface, LeFort III (extra and intracranial) with forehead advancement (eg, mono bloc), requiring bone grafts (includes obtaining autografts); without LeFort I
	See current CPT manual for possible additional procedure codes.
Available Medical Diagnosis Code(s) - ICD-9-CM **(International Classification of Diseases-9th Revision-Clinical Modification)**	
524.02	Maxillary hyperplasia
524.11	Maxillary asymmetry
	See ICD-9-CM for possible additional diagnosis codes.

Dental Procedure Code	
(Code on Dental Procedures and Nomenclature)	
D7950	osseous, osteoperiosteal, or cartilage graft of the mandible or maxilla - autogenous or nonautogenous, by report
Available Medical Procedure Code(s) – CPT	
(Current Procedure Terminology)	
20900	Bone graft, any donor area; minor or small (eg, dowel or button)
20902	Bone graft, any donor area: major or large
21125	Augmentation, mandibular body or angle; prosthetic material
21299	Unlisted craniofacial and maxillofacial procedure (Note: Include narrative that explains circumstances and describes procedure.)
	See current CPT manual for possible additional procedure codes.
Available Medical Diagnosis Code(s) - ICD-9-CM	
(International Classification of Diseases-9th Revision-Clinical Modification)	
525.23	Severe atrophy of the mandible
526.89	Disease, jaw NEC
	See ICD-9-CM for possible additional diagnosis codes.

. . .

Dental Procedure Code	
(Code on Dental Procedures and Nomenclature)	
D7951	sinus augmentation with bone or bone substitutes
Available Medical Procedure Code(s) – CPT	
(Current Procedure Terminology)	
21299	Unlisted craniofacial and maxillofacial procedure (Note: Include narrative that explains circumstances and describes procedure.)
Available Medical Diagnosis Code(s) - ICD-9-CM	
(International Classification of Diseases-9th Revision-Clinical Modification)	
525.25	Moderate atrophy of maxilla
525.26	Severe atrophy of maxilla
	See ICD-9-CM for possible additional diagnosis codes.

Dental Procedure Code *(Code on Dental Procedures and Nomenclature)*	
D7953	bone replacement graft for ridge preservation – per site
Available Medical Procedure Code(s) – CPT (Current Procedure Terminology)	
20900	Bone graft, any donor area; minor or small (eg, dowel or button)
21299	Unlisted craniofacial and maxillofacial procedure (Note: Include narrative that explains circumstances and describes procedure.)
Available Medical Diagnosis Code(s) - ICD-9-CM (International Classification of Diseases-9th Revision-Clinical Modification)	
525.12	Loss of teeth due to periodontal disease
525.13	Loss of teeth due to caries
	See ICD-9-CM Section 520 - 529 (Diseases of Oral Cavity, Salivary Glands, and Jaws) for possible additional diagnosis codes.

. . .

Dental Procedure Code *(Code on Dental Procedures and Nomenclature)*	
D7955	repair of maxillofacial soft and/or hard tissue defect
Available Medical Procedure Code(s) – CPT (Current Procedure Terminology)	
40702	Plastic repair of cleft lip/nasal deformity; primary bilateral, one of two stages
21299	Unlisted craniofacial and maxillofacial procedure (Note: Include narrative that explains circumstances and describes procedure.)
	See current CPT manual for possible additional procedure codes.
Available Medical Diagnosis Code(s) - ICD-9-CM (International Classification of Diseases-9th Revision-Clinical Modification)	
749.03	Cleft palate and lip bilateral complete
749.13	Cleft lip, bilateral complete
	See ICD-9-CM for possible additional diagnosis codes.

Dental Procedure Code *(Code on Dental Procedures and Nomenclature)*	
D7960	frenulectomy - also known as frenectomy or frenotomy - separate procedure not incidental to another procedure
D7963	frenuloplasty
Available Medical Procedure Code(s) – CPT (Current Procedure Terminology)	
41010	Incision of lingual frenum (frenotomy)
41115	Excision of lingual frenum (frenectomy)
41520	Frenuloplasty (surgical revision of frenum, eg, with Z-plasty)
	See current CPT manual for possible additional procedure codes.
Available Medical Diagnosis Code(s) - ICD-9-CM (International Classification of Diseases-9th Revision-Clinical Modification)	
524.59	Other dentofacial functional abnormalities
750.0	Tongue tie, congenital
	See ICD-9-CM for possible additional diagnosis codes.

. . .

Dental Procedure Code *(Code on Dental Procedures and Nomenclature)*	
D7970	excision of hyperplastic tissue - per arch
Available Medical Procedure Code(s) – CPT (Current Procedure Terminology)	
41828	Excision of hyperplastic alveolar mucosa, each quadrant (specify)
	See current CPT manual for possible additional procedure codes.
Available Medical Diagnosis Code(s) - ICD-9-CM (International Classification of Diseases-9th Revision-Clinical Modification)	
528.6	Leukoplakia of oral mucosa (gingiva)
528.79	Other disturbances of oral epithelium, including tongue
	See ICD-9-CM for possible additional diagnosis codes.

Dental Procedure Code (Code on Dental Procedures and Nomenclature)	
D7971	excision of pericoronal gingiva
Available Medical Procedure Code(s) – CPT (Current Procedure Terminology)	
41821	Operculectomy, excision pericoronal tissue
	See current CPT manual for possible additional procedure codes.
Available Medical Diagnosis Code(s) - ICD-9-CM (International Classification of Diseases-9th Revision-Clinical Modification)	
523.11	Chronic gingivitis, non-plaque induced
	See ICD-9-CM Section 520 - 529 (Diseases of Oral Cavity, Salivary Glands, and Jaws) for possible additional diagnosis codes.

. . .

Dental Procedure Code (Code on Dental Procedures and Nomenclature)	
D7972	surgical reduction of fibrous tuberosity
Available Medical Procedure Code(s) – CPT (Current Procedure Terminology)	
41822	Excision of fibrous tuberosities, dentoalveolar structures
	See current CPT manual for possible additional procedure codes.
Available Medical Diagnosis Code(s) - ICD-9-CM (International Classification of Diseases-9th Revision-Clinical Modification)	
528.8	Oral submucosal fibrosis of the oral soft tissue
	See ICD-9-CM for possible additional diagnosis codes.

Dental Procedure Code	
(Code on Dental Procedures and Nomenclature)	
D7980	sialolithotomy
Available Medical Procedure Code(s) – CPT	
(Current Procedure Terminology)	
42330	Sialolithotomy; submandibular (submaxillary), sublingual or parotid, uncomplicated, intraoral
42335	Sialolithotomy; submandibular (submaxillary), complicated, intraoral
42340	Sialolithotomy; parotid, extraoral or complicated intraoral
	See current CPT manual for possible additional procedure codes.
Available Medical Diagnosis Code(s) - ICD-9-CM	
(International Classification of Diseases-9th Revision-Clinical Modification)	
527.2	Sialoadentitis
527.4	Fistula, salivary gland
	See ICD-9-CM for possible additional diagnosis codes.

. . .

Dental Procedure Code	
(Code on Dental Procedures and Nomenclature)	
D7981	excision of salivary gland, by report
Available Medical Procedure Code(s) – CPT	
(Current Procedure Terminology)	
42440	Excision of submandibular (submaxillary) gland
42450	Excision of sublingual gland
	See current CPT manual for possible additional procedure codes.
Available Medical Diagnosis Code(s) - ICD-9-CM	
(International Classification of Diseases-9th Revision-Clinical Modification)	
142.1	Neoplasm, malignant, submandibular gland
210.2	Neoplasm, benign, sublingual gland
527.9	Disease, salivary gland NOS
	See ICD-9-CM for possible additional diagnosis codes.

Dental Procedure Code
(Code on Dental Procedures and Nomenclature)

D7982	sialodochoplasty

Available Medical Procedure Code(s) – CPT
(Current Procedure Terminology)

42500	Plastic repair of salivary duct, sialodochoplasty; primary or simple
42505	Plastic repair of salivary duct, sialodochoplasty; secondary or complicated
	See current CPT manual for possible additional procedure codes.

Available Medical Diagnosis Code(s) - ICD-9-CM
(International Classification of Diseases-9th Revision-Clinical Modification)

527.1	Hypertrophy, salivary gland
527.5	Sialolithiasis
	See ICD-9-CM for possible additional diagnosis codes.

. . .

Dental Procedure Code
(Code on Dental Procedures and Nomenclature)

D7983	closure of salivary fistula

Available Medical Procedure Code(s) – CPT
(Current Procedure Terminology)

42600	Closure salivary fistula

Available Medical Diagnosis Code(s) - ICD-9-CM
(International Classification of Diseases-9th Revision-Clinical Modification)

527.4	Fistula, salivary gland
527.6	Mucocele, salivary gland
	See ICD-9-CM Section 520 - 529 (Diseases of Oral Cavity, Salivary Glands, and Jaws) for possible additional diagnosis codes.

Dental Procedure Code *(Code on Dental Procedures and Nomenclature)*	
D7990	emergency tracheotomy
Available Medical Procedure Code(s) – CPT **(Current Procedure Terminology)**	
31603	Tracheostomy, emergency procedure; transtracheal
31605	Tracheostomy, emergency procedure; cricothyroid membrane
Available Medical Diagnosis Code(s) - ICD-9-CM **(International Classification of Diseases-9th Revision-Clinical Modification)**	
799.0	Asphyxia
933.1	Foreign body in larynx
	See ICD-9-CM for possible additional diagnosis codes.

· · ·

Dental Procedure Code *(Code on Dental Procedures and Nomenclature)*	
D7991	coronoidectomy
Available Medical Procedure Code(s) – CPT **(Current Procedure Terminology)**	
21070	Coronoidectomy (separate procedure)
Available Medical Diagnosis Code(s) - ICD-9-CM **(International Classification of Diseases-9th Revision-Clinical Modification)**	
802.23	Fracture, coronoid process, mandible, closed
802.33	Fracture, coronoid process, mandible, open
	See ICD-9-CM for possible additional diagnosis codes.

Dental Procedure Code
(Code on Dental Procedures and Nomenclature)

D7995	synthetic graft - mandible or facial bones, by report

Available Medical Procedure Code(s) – CPT
(Current Procedure Terminology)

21299	Unlisted craniofacial and maxillofacial procedure (Note: Include narrative that explains circumstances and describes procedure.)

Available Medical Diagnosis Code(s) - ICD-9-CM
(International Classification of Diseases-9th Revision-Clinical Modification)

524.04	Mandibular hypoplasia
	See ICD-9-CM for possible additional diagnosis codes.

. . .

Dental Procedure Code
(Code on Dental Procedures and Nomenclature)

D7996	implant-mandible for augmentation purposes (excluding alveolar ridge), by report

Available Medical Procedure Code(s) – CPT
(Current Procedure Terminology)

21299	Unlisted craniofacial and maxillofacial procedure (Note: Include narrative that explains circumstances and describes procedure.)

Available Medical Diagnosis Code(s) - ICD-9-CM
(International Classification of Diseases-9th Revision-Clinical Modification)

754.0	Deformity, skull / face / jaw, congenital
	See ICD-9-CM for possible additional diagnosis codes.

Dental Procedure Code
(Code on Dental Procedures and Nomenclature)
D7997   appliance removal (not by dentist who placed appliance), includes removal of archbar

Available Medical Procedure Code(s) – CPT
(Current Procedure Terminology)
20694   Removal, under anesthesia, of external fixation system
20670   Removal of implant; superficial (eg, buried wire, pin or rod) (separate procedure)
20680   Removal of implant; deep (eg, buried wire, pin, screw, metal band, nail, rod or plate)
See current CPT manual for possible additional procedure codes.

Available Medical Diagnosis Code(s) - ICD-9-CM
(International Classification of Diseases-9th Revision-Clinical Modification)
802.25   Fracture, mandible, closed, angle of jaw
802.35   Fracture, mandible, open, angle of jaw
See ICD-9-CM for possible additional diagnosis codes.

. . .

Dental Procedure Code
(Code on Dental Procedures and Nomenclature)
D7998   intraoral placement of a fixation device not in conjunction with a fracture

Available Medical Procedure Code(s) – CPT
(Current Procedure Terminology)
21110   Application of interdental fixation device for conditions other than fracture or dislocation, includes removal
21497   Interdental wiring, for condition other than fracture
See current CPT manual for possible additional procedure codes.

Available Medical Diagnosis Code(s) - ICD-9-CM
(International Classification of Diseases-9th Revision-Clinical Modification)
525.20   Unspecified atrophy of edentulous alveolar ridge
See ICD-9-CM for possible additional diagnosis codes.

VII. Adjunctive General Services

Dental Procedure Code *(Code on Dental Procedures and Nomenclature)*	
D9212	regional block anesthesia
Available Medical Procedure Code(s) – CPT **(Current Procedure Terminology)**	
64400	Injection, anesthetic agent; trigeminal nerve, any division or branch
	See current CPT manual for possible additional procedure codes.
Available Medical Diagnosis Code(s) - ICD-9-CM **(International Classification of Diseases-9th Revision-Clinical Modification)**	
350.1	Neuralgia, trigeminal
350.2	Pain, atypical face
524.64	Disorder, TMJ, joint sounds on opening and/or closing the jaw
	See ICD-9-CM for possible additional diagnosis codes.

. . .

Dental Procedure Code *(Code on Dental Procedures and Nomenclature)*	
D9220	deep sedation/general anesthesia – first 30 minutes
D9221	deep sedation/general anesthesia - each additional 15 minutes
Available Medical Procedure Code(s) – CPT **(Current Procedure Terminology)**	
00170	Anesthesia for intraoral procedures, including biopsy; not otherwise specified
	See current CPT manual for possible additional procedure codes.
Available Medical Diagnosis Code(s) - ICD-9-CM **(International Classification of Diseases-9th Revision-Clinical Modification)**	
520.6	Disturbances of tooth eruption
802.25	Fracture of face bones: angle of jaw
	See ICD-9-CM for possible additional diagnosis codes.

Dental Procedure Code *(Code on Dental Procedures and Nomenclature)*	
D9241	intravenous conscious sedation/analgesia – first 30 minutes
D9242	intravenous conscious sedation/analgesia – each additional 15 minutes
Available Medical Procedure Code(s) – CPT (Current Procedure Terminology)	
	See Moderate (Conscious) Sedation guidelines and codes 99143-99150 in the current CPT manual for these procedures.
Available Medical Diagnosis Code(s) - ICD-9-CM (International Classification of Diseases-9th Revision-Clinical Modification)	
520.6	Disturbances of tooth eruption
802.25	Fracture of face bones: angle of jaw
	See ICD-9-CM for possible additional diagnosis codes.

Dental Procedure Code *(Code on Dental Procedures and Nomenclature)*

D9310	consultation – diagnostic service provided by dentist or physician other than requesting dentist or physician

Available Medical Procedure Code(s) – CPT **(Current Procedure Terminology)**

99241	Office consultation for a new or established patient, which requires these 3 key components: • A problem focused history; • A problem focused examination; and • Straightforward medical decision making Counseling and/or coordination of care with other providers or agencies are provided consistent with the nature of the problem(s) and the patient's and/or family's needs. Usually, the presenting problem(s) are self limited or minor. Physicians typically spend 15 minutes face-to-face with the patient and/or family.
99242	Office consultation for a new or established patient, which requires these 3 key components: • An expanded problem focused history; • An expanded problem focused examination; and • Straightforward medical decision making Counseling and/or coordination of care with other providers or agencies are provided consistent with the nature of the problem(s) and the patient's and/or family's needs. Usually, the presenting problem(s) are of low severity. Physicians typically spend 30 minutes face-to-face with the patient and/or family. See current CPT manual for possible additional Evaluation and Management consultation procedure codes (eg, 99243-99245).

Available Medical Diagnosis Code(s) - ICD-9-CM **(International Classification of Diseases-9th Revision-Clinical Modification)**

	See ICD-9-CM for possible diagnosis codes.

HIPAA
Overview

11 CDT
Companion

ADA American Dental Association®
America's leading advocate for oral health

Chapter 11
HIPAA Overview

On August 21, 1996 the Health Insurance Portability and Accountability Act of 1996 (HIPAA), P.L. 104-191, was signed into law. The Portability portion of the law, which was designed to maintain health insurance coverage for employees when they change employers, was put into effect immediately.

Administrative Simplification provisions of the law, put into effect over time, address standards for the electronic transmission of health information, and the privacy and security of that information. These provisions are intended to reduce the costs and administrative burdens of health care by making it possible to electronically transmit, using standard formats and content, certain administrative and financial transactions that are often prepared and processed manually using proprietary paper forms.

Rationale for HIPAA Administrative Simplification and Standard Transactions

An unjustifiably high percentage of every health care dollar is spent on administrative overhead. Administrative overhead includes processes for:
- enrolling an individual in a health plan;
- paying health insurance premiums;
- checking insurance eligibility for a particular service;
- getting an authorization to refer a patient to a specialist;
- filing a claim for payment for health care that has been delivered;
- requesting or responding to additional information in support of a claim;
- coordinating the payment of a claim involving two or more insurance companies; and
- notifying the provider about the payment of a claim.[1]

Without automation, these processes involve numerous paper forms and telephone calls. In addition, there are many delays in communicating information among different locations, which creates problems and increased costs for health care providers, plans and insurers alike.

To address these problems, the health care industry attempted to develop standards for accomplishing these transactions electronically. However, it was difficult to get all participants to voluntarily agree to follow a single, uniform set of standards. Consequently, Congress included the Administrative Simplification provisions in HIPAA. To address concerns about the potential for abuse of electronic access to this type of information, the law also includes specific provisions to protect the security and confidentiality of health information that might be associated with an individual.

[1] Centers for Medicare and Medicaid Services, Health Insurance Portability and Accountability Act of 1996, "Implementation of Administrative Simplification Requirements by HHS." http://aspe.hhs.gov/admnsimp/kkimpl.htm.

The HIPAA standards apply to the following transactions:

- health care claims or equivalent encounter information
- health care payment and remittance advice
- coordination of benefits
- health care claim status
- enrollment and disenrollment in a health plan
- eligibility for a health plan
- health plan premium payments
- referral certification and authorization
- first report of injury
- health claims attachments
- other transactions that the secretary may prescribe by regulation

The law requires health plans to be able to accept standard electronic transactions from health care providers. However the law places no mandate on dentists or other health care providers to submit claims electronically. Should a health care provider wish to conduct these transactions electronically a HIPAA standard transaction must be used.

The *Code* as a HIPAA Administrative Simplification Standard

On August 17, 2000, the Department of Health and Human Services (HHS) named the ADA's *Code on Dental Procedures and Nomenclature (Code)* as the national standard code set for dental procedures to be used on electronic dental claims. This was done under the authority of the Health Insurance Portability and Accountability Act of 1996 (HIPAA). All third-party payers that accept electronic claims must use procedure codes that are in effect on the date of service submitted, in order to be compliant with HIPAA.

Why is that important to you? When you submit a procedure code that has been deleted on the date the procedure is performed, your claim will be rejected. Delays in processing cause frustration for payers, patients and providers.

The current version of the paper claim form harmonizes its data content with the HIPAA standard electronic dental claim. The internal processing policies of payers are merging electronic and paper claims, so current codes are needed on paper claims as well.

If you are asked whether HIPAA requires the use of current codes for paper claims, the short answer is HIPAA does not affect paper claim forms. However, payers are expecting the current version of the *Code*, since all claims go into the same claims adjudication system; and there may be state regulations that apply to this question.

Current and Upcoming HIPAA Standard Transactions

The current HIPAA standard electronic dental claim transaction is version 4010. In 2009 the secretary of HHS published a notice in the Federal Register that a new version of this HIPAA standard transaction (and for others currently in use such as the medical benefit claim) will become effective January 1, 2012. This is version 5010 that incorporates changes that may affect how you prepare and submit electronic claims. These changes include recognition of the ICD-9-CM diagnosis code set for possible use in a HIPAA electronic claim – and use of ICD-10-CM as of January 1. 2013.

Please contact your practice management system vendor to determine what actions may be necessary to ensure your ability to continue efficient electronic claim submission.

Compliance Rules – Use of Standard Transactions by Payers, Dentists and other Health Care Community Members

Health plans, payers, and clearinghouses must be able to send or receive the designated transactions in the standard electronic form no later than 24 months after the secretary adopts the standard (36 months for small plans). Those that cannot perform these standard electronic transactions may comply by contracting with a clearinghouse to perform them. However, the responsibility for compliance remains with the primary entity.

Dentists and other health care providers who elect to exchange information electronically must use a HIPAA standard electronic transaction when one is available HIPAA recognizes and permits dentists and other health care providers to contract with a clearinghouse when necessary to prepare and transmit, or receive on their behalf, the standard transactions.

When employers act in the role of a health plan or a health care provider, they too must comply with the standards and may contract with a clearinghouse or third-party administrator to conduct the standard transactions for them.

Health plans may not refuse to accept standard transactions submitted electronically (on their own or through clearinghouses). Further, health plans may not delay payment because the transactions are submitted electronically in compliance with the standards.

The following exceptions exist:

Nonstandard transactions. The standards for the designated transactions apply when those transactions are transmitted electronically but not to transactions conducted by paper, telephone, or personal interactive systems. Individual payers such as Medicare elected to extend the standard requirements to include paper-based transactions. However, this is not required by HIPAA.

Transmissions within corporate entities. Clearly, electronic transmission of any of the specified transactions between corporate entities must comply with the standards adopted by the secretary. However, transmissions of these transactions within a corporate entity are not required to comply with the standards. For example, a hospital that is wholly owned by a managed care company would not have to use the standards to pass encounter information back to the home office; it would have to use the standard claim transaction to submit a claim to another payer.

Workers' compensation. The HIPAA definition of a health plan does not specifically include workers' compensation programs or carriers. However, the list of designated transactions for which the secretary must adopt standards for electronic transmission includes First Report of Injury, which is the primary transaction used to initiate workers' compensation actions. For this reason, the secretary will be proposing a standard for First Report of Injury and will be considering different ways of achieving compliance with this standard.

Health plan sponsors. Health plan sponsors, including employers when they act in the role of a sponsor, are not covered explicitly by the law but may benefit from the adoption of standards and electronic transactions. Sponsors may elect to use standard enrollment, disenrollment, and premium payment transactions, which must be accepted by all health plans when submitted electronically. Market forces may move health plans to require sponsors to use the standards for electronic transactions, although this is not mandated by the law.

[2] Centers for Medicare and Medicaid Services, Health Insurance Portability and Accountability Act of 1996, "Implementation of Administrative Simplification Requirements by HHS." http://aspe.hhs.gov/admnsimp/kkimpl.htm.

Compliance Rules – Electronic Media Transmissions

All electronic transmissions of the specified transactions from one computer to another must comply with the standards. Electronic transmissions include all media, such as magnetic tape, disk, or CD. Transmissions over the Internet, intranets, leased lines, dial-up lines, private networks, etc, are all included. Telephone voice response and faxback systems would not be included. The Hyper Text Markup Language (HTML) interaction between a server and a browser by which the elements of a transaction are solicited from a user would not be included. However, once assembled into a transaction by the server, transmission of the full transaction to another corporate entity, such as a payer, must comply.

The only exception involves the use of clearinghouses as described here:

- Dentists and other health care providers may submit nonstandard transactions to clearinghouses, which must convert the data into the standard transaction before forwarding it on to the payer.

- Payers may submit nonstandard transactions to clearinghouses, which must also create the standard transaction before forwarding it on to the health care provider.

- A clearinghouse may convert standard transactions into paper or other nonstandard format for receipt by a health care provider or plan that does not have the capacity to receive such transactions in standard format.

Other HIPAA Administrative Simplification Requirements

Privacy
The privacy requirements limit the release of patient protected health information (PHI) without the patient's knowledge and consent beyond that required for patient care. Patient's personal information must be more securely guarded and more carefully handled when conducting the business of health care.[3] The ADA HIPAA Privacy Kit can be obtained through the ADA Catalog at **http://www.adacatalog.org**.

Security
The Security Regulation outlines the minimum administrative, technical, and physical safeguards required to prevent unauthorized access to protected health care information. The ADA HIPAA Security Kit can be obtained through the ADA Catalog at http://www.adacatalog.org.

National Identifiers
HIPAA will require that health care providers, health plans, and employers have standard national numbers that identify them on standard transactions. *(For further information on the National Provider Identifier, go to Chapter 7 - Dental Claim Submission)*

Additional information on HIPAA is available at www.ada.org/goto/hipaa.

---

[3] HIPAA Administrative Simplification — HIPAA Information Series for Providers, Volume 1, Paper 1, http://www.cms.gov/EducationMaterials/Downloads/HIPAA101-1.pdf

Commonly Used Acronyms Concerning Dental Care, Benefit Administration and Electronic Commerce

12

CDT
Companion

Chapter 12
Commonly Used Acronyms Concerning Dental Care, Benefit Administration and Electronic Commerce

While reading this and other publications, and as you increase your involvement with electronic transactions, you may run into one or many of the acronyms listed below. The ADA recommends that where an internet address is provided, you should link to that Web site for the most current information.

AHIMA   **American Health Information Management Association**
AHIMA is an association of health information management (HIM) professionals. AHIMA's members are dedicated to the management of personal health information needed to deliver quality healthcare to the public. Founded in 1928 to improve the quality of medical records, AHIMA is committed to advancing the HIM profession in an increasingly electronic and global environment through leadership in advocacy, education, certification, and lifelong learning.
www.ahima.org

AHIP   **America's Health Insurance Plans**
AHIP is the national association representing nearly 1,300 member companies providing health insurance coverage to more than 200 million Americans. These companies offer medical expense insurance, long-term care insurance, disability income insurance, dental insurance, supplemental insurance, stop-loss insurance and reinsurance to consumers, employers, and public purchasers. AHIP's goal is to provide a unified voice for the health care financing industry, to expand access to high quality, cost effective health care to all Americans, and to ensure Americans' financial security through robust insurance markets, product flexibility and innovation, and an abundance of consumer choice.
www.ahip.org

AHRQ   **Agency for Healthcare Research and Quality (formerly AHCPR)**
An agency that is part of the U.S. Department of Health and Human Services, and is the lead agency charged with supporting research designed to improve the quality of healthcare, reduce its cost, improve patient safety, decrease medical errors, and broaden access to essential services. AHRQ sponsors and conducts research that provides evidence-based information on healthcare outcomes; quality; and cost, use, and access. The information helps healthcare decision makers — patients and clinicians, health system leaders, and policymakers — make more informed decisions and improve the quality of healthcare services.
www.ahrq.gov

ANSI   **American National Standards Institute**
Founded in 1918, ANSI is a private, non-profit organization (501(c) 3) that administers and coordinates the U.S. voluntary standardization and conformity assessment system. ANSI's mission is to enhance both the global competitiveness of U.S. business and the U.S. quality of life by promoting and facilitating voluntary consensus standards and conformity assessment systems, and safeguarding their integrity.
www.ansi.org

ASC   **Accredited Standards Committee**
A body that develops standards in accordance with a consensus process accredited by ANSI. (see ANSI)

ANSI   **American National Standards Institute Accredited Standards Committee X12 ASC X12N   Insurance Subcommittee**
The ANSI accredited SDO that creates EDI transactions for various sectors of the business community, including Health Care. Several X12 transactions have been named as HIPAA standards. X12N is subcommittee that creates insurance EDI transaction standards.

www.X12.org (from the "Committees/Groups" drop-down menu select Subcommittees then Insurance)

ASO   **Administrative Services Only**
A service offered by third-party payers, or third-party administrators, to manage a self-insured benefit plan on behalf of an employer group or other entity offering dental or medical benefits. In some situations a third-party payer may also provide risk-based 'stop-loss' coverage on top of the self-insured program.

BC/BS **Blue Cross and Blue Shield Plans**
Independent third-party payers that have agreed to provide health care benefit programs on a local basis using the Blue Cross and Blue Shield name and service marks. Each Plan may use the name and marks in specific service areas. There are inter-plan agreements that enable delivery of benefits on a national basis. (See BCBSA)

BCBSA **Blue Cross and Blue Shield Association**
The national association of independent BC and BS Plans that licenses use of the Blue Cross and Blue Shield names and service marks.
www.bcbsa.com

CAP **College of American Pathologists**
The professional association that established SNOMED (See SNOMED). In November 2005 CAP's SNOMED International Division announced transfer of development, ownership and maintenance of SNOMED to an Executive Agency of the Department of Health in England, which would establish an International Standards Development Organization (SDO) for such activity. (See SNOMED)

CDBP **Council on Dental Benefit Programs**
The Council on Dental Benefit Programs is the ADA agency dedicated to promoting quality dental care through the development, promotion and monitoring of dental benefit programs for the public, as well as by development and maintenance of coding taxonomies and quality assessment and improvement tools and methodologies.

CDT **Current Dental Terminology**
This acronym is sometimes used as the name for the *Code on Dental Procedures and Nomenclature*. CDT is the ADA manual which contains the *Code on Dental Procedures and Nomenclature* and other information concerning procedure documentation and claim submission.

CHAMPUS **Civilian Health and Medical Program of the Uniformed Services**
See Tricare

CHIP **Children's Health Insurance Program/Medicare-Medicaid**
See SCHIP

CMS **Centers for Medicare and Medicaid Services (federal agency; prior name – HCFA)**
A Federal agency within the Department of Health and Human Services (HHS) whose mission is to assure health care security for beneficiaries covered by Medicare and Medicaid programs. CMS also is the lead agency on HIPAA and health care electronic commerce activity through its Office of E-Health Standards and Services (OESS).
www.cms.gov

CRC   **Code Revision Committee**
The body responsible for determining revisions to the *Code on Dental Procedures and Nomenclature*. There are twelve voting members on the CRC, evenly balanced between dentistry's practitioner and payer sectors. The six ADA representatives are nominated by the Council on Dental Benefit Programs and appointed by the ADA President.
www.ada.org/goto/dentalcode

DBIS   **Dental Benefit Information Service and Third Party Issues**
The Council on Dental Benefit Programs Subcommittee that was established as the authority and primary resource for plan sponsors and patients in need of assistance in designing effective dental benefit plans. The goals of DBIS are to promote fee-for-service, freedom of choice dental benefit plans; promote Direct Reimbursement (DR) to plan purchasers via the national DR marketing campaign and monitor trends and offer information on all types of dental benefits. The third-party issues staff provides assistance direct to members and their staff who have questions and concerns with third-party payers.
www.ada.org/goto/dr

DCC   **Data Content Committee**
A term used in HIPAA regulations that denotes bodies whose mission includes establishing the business needs for standard transactions (electronic or paper, as applicable) within the health care community. There are three DCC's identified under HIPAA, the National Uniform Billing Committee, the National Uniform Claim Committee, and the Dental Content Committee.

DDPA   **Delta Dental Plans Association**
A not-for-profit organization, with some for-profit affiliates, that offers a nationwide system of dental health benefits for a wide range of employers.
www.deltadental.com

DeCC   **Dental Content Committee**
The DeCC is the deliberative body sponsored and chaired by the ADA that has been established in accordance with the administrative simplification provisions of the HIPAA to cooperate in the maintenance of the standards adopted under HIPAA. It has been named as a Designated Standards Maintenance Organization (DSMO) by the Secretary of the Department of Health and Human Services. As such, the DeCC addresses standard transaction content on behalf of the dental sector of the health care community.
www.ada.org/goto/decc

DHMOs **Dental Health Maintenance Organizations**
The equivalent of a medical Health Maintenance Organization for dentistry.

DICOM **Dental Imaging and Communication in Medicine**
An ANSI ASC whose standard for medical imaging is recognized by the ADA and the Association is a DICOM member. The DICOM standard enables systems used in medical imaging to be interoperable.
http://medical.nema.org

DPPC **Dental Practice Parameters Committee**
The ADA began a program to develop practice parameters in 1989. During the 1993 House of Delegates, the ADA House approved a parameters development process and created the Dental Practice Parameters Committee. The DPPC has drafted proposed parameters, and at its 1994 annual session, the ADA House of Delegates approved parameters for 12 dental conditions.

DR **Direct Reimbursement**
Direct reimbursement is a self-funded program in which the individual is reimbursed based on a percentage of dollars spent for dental care provided, and which allows beneficiaries to seek treatment from the dentist of their choice.
www.ada.org/goto/dr

DSMO **Designated Standards Maintenance Organization**
The final HIPAA rule titled "Standards for Electronic Transactions," published in the Federal Register on August 17, 2000, establishes a new category of organization, the "Designated Standard Maintenance Organization (DSMO)." Section 162.910 of this final regulation provides that the Secretary may designate as DSMOs those organizations that agree to maintain the standards adopted by the Secretary. Several Data Content Committees (DCCs) and Standard Setting Organizations (SSOs) have agreed to maintain those standards. (See DCC and SDO)

EDI **Electronic Data Interchange**
The transfer of data between different companies using networks, such as Value Added Networks (VANS) or the Internet. ANSI has approved a set of EDI standards known as the X12 standards.

EHNAC **Electronic Healthcare Network Accreditation Commission**
EHNAC was established by health care industry participants as an independent, not-for-profit accrediting body. It establishes criteria for measuring the performance of clearinghouses and value-added networks.
www.ehnac.org

EOB

Explanation of Benefits

A written statement to a beneficiary, from a third-party payer, after a claim has been reported, indicating the benefit/charges covered or not covered by the dental benefits plan.

ERISA

Employee Retirement Income Security Act of 1974

ERISA is a federal law that sets minimum standards for most voluntarily established pension and health plans in private industry to provide protection for individuals in these plans.

HCFA

Health Care Financing Administration – (obsolete name; See CMS)

HCPCS

Healthcare Common Procedure Coding System

A code set recognized for use in HIPAA standard transactions. HCPCS is divided into two principal subsystems, referred to as level I and level II. Level I is comprised of CPT (Current Procedural Terminology), a numeric coding system maintained by the American Medical Association (AMA). Level II is a standardized coding system that is used primarily to identify products, supplies, and services not included in the CPT codes. The *Code on Dental Procedures and Nomenclature* is listed in HCPCS as Level II "D" codes under an agreement between the ADA and CMS.

www.cms.hhs.gov/MedHCPCSGenInfo

HEDIS

Health Plan Employer Data & Information Set

A set of measures that are used to report the performance of health plans. The measures evaluate the organizational structure and systems of the HMO and the performance in delivering care. HEDIS was created by the National Committee for Quality Assurance (See NCQA).

HHS

Department of Health and Human Services

HHS is the United States government's principal agency for protecting the health of all Americans and providing essential human services, especially for those who are least able to help themselves. The Department includes more than three hundred programs covering a wide spectrum of activities. HHS-funded services are provided at the local level by state or county agencies, or through private sector grantees. The Department's programs are administered by 11 operating divisions, including eight agencies in the U.S. Public Health Service and three human services agencies. CMS is one of HHS' major agencies.

www.hhs.gov

HIPAA

Health Insurance Portability and Accountability Act of 1996

Federal legislation whose two major parts address 1) portability of health care benefits by employees, and 2) reduction in heath care administrative costs through adoption of standard electronic administrative and financial transactions, including the means to ensure the security and privacy of such information.

HIPDB **Healthcare Integrity & Protection Data Bank**

The Secretary, HHS acting through the Office of Inspector General (OIG) was directed by HIPAA to create HIPDB to combat fraud and abuse in health insurance and health care delivery. HIPDB is primarily a flagging system that may serve to alert users that a comprehensive review of a practitioner's, provider's, or supplier's past actions may be prudent. The data bank is intended to augment, not replace, traditional forms of review and investigation, serving as an important supplement to a careful review of a practitioner's, provider's, or supplier's past actions.
www.npdb-hipdb.com

HITSP **Healthcare Information Technology Standards Panel**

HITSP's mission is to serve as a cooperative partnership between the public and private sectors for the purpose of achieving a widely accepted and useful set of standards specifically to enable and support widespread interoperability among healthcare software applications, as they will interact in a local, regional and national health information network for the United States. The Panel will assist in the development of the U.S. Nationwide Health Information Network (NHIN) by addressing issues such as privacy and security within a shared healthcare information system. HITSP is sponsored by the American National Standards Institute (See ANSI).

HL7 **Health Level 7**

The ANSI accredited SDO that creates develops messaging standards that enable disparate healthcare applications to exchange keys sets of clinical and administrative data. HL7 standards are referenced in the pending HIPAA regulation concerning claim attachments.
www.hl7.org

IG **Implementation Guide**

Technical specifications for implementation of a HIPAA electronic transaction. An obsolete term. (See "TR3")

ISO **International Organization for Standardization (ISO is the abbreviation en Francais)**

ISO is a worldwide federation of national standards bodies, one in each country. The organization's objective is to promote the development of standardization and related activities in the world with a view to facilitating international exchange of goods and services, and to developing cooperation in the spheres of intellectual, scientific, technological and economic activity. The results of ISO technical work are published as International Standards.
www.iso.org

JCAHO   **Joint Commission on the Accreditation of Healthcare Organizations**
The JCHAO mission is to continuously improve the safety and quality of care provided to the public through the provision of health care accreditation and related services that support performance improvement in health care organizations.
www.jointcommission.org

LEAT   **Least Expensive Alternative Treatment**
A limitation in a dental benefit plan that will only allow benefits for the least expensive treatment. Also referred to as Least Expensive Professionally Acceptable Alternative Treatment (LEPAAT).

NADP   **National Association of Dental Plans**
NADP is a non-profit trade association representing the entire dental benefits industry, i.e. dental HMOs, dental PPOs, discount dental plans and dental indemnity products. These member dental plans provide dental benefits to 107 million of the 159 million Americans with dental benefits, i.e. 67% of the total dental benefits market. Member organizations include major commercial carriers, regional and single state companies, as well as companies organized as Delta and Blue Cross Blue Shield plans.
www.nadp.org

NAIC   **National Association of Insurance Commissioners**
The mission of the NAIC is to assist state insurance regulators, individually and collectively, in serving the public interest and achieving the following fundamental insurance regulatory goals in a responsive, efficient and cost effective manner, consistent with the wishes of its members:
www.naic.org

NCPDP   **National Council for Prescription Drug Programs**
NCPDP creates and promotes standards for the transfer of data to and from the pharmacy services sector of the healthcare industry. The organization provides a forum and support wherein our diverse membership can efficiently and effectively develop and maintain these standards through a consensus building process. The NCPDP retail pharmacy claim transaction (5.1) is a named HIPAA standard.
www.ncpdp.org

NCQA   **National Committee on Quality Assurance**
NCQA's mission is to improve the quality of health care. Its vision is to transform health care quality through measurement, transparency and accountability.
www.ncqa.org

NCVHS   **National Committee on Vital and Health Statistics**
The NCVHS was established by Congress to serve as an advisory body to the Department of Health and Human Services on health data, statistics and national health information policy. It fulfills important review and advisory functions relative to health data and statistical problems of national and international interest, stimulates or conducts studies of such problems and makes proposals for improvement of the Nation's health statistics and information systems. In 1996, the Committee was restructured to meet expanded responsibilities under the Health Insurance Portability and Accountability Act of 1996 (HIPAA).
www.ncvhs.hhs.gov

NDEDIC   **National Dental Electronic Data Interchange Council**
NDEDIC is an organization that unites all stakeholders in the dental industry to promote electronic commerce, providing a unified forum for dental EDI. The ADA is an NDEDIC member.
www.ndedic.com/home

NPDB   **National Practitioner Data Bank**
The NPDB is primarily an alert or flagging system intended to facilitate a comprehensive review of health care practitioners' professional credentials. The information contained in the NPDB is intended to direct discrete inquiry into, and scrutiny of, specific areas of a practitioner's licensure, professional society memberships, medical malpractice payment history, and record of clinical privileges.
www.npdb-hipdb.com

NPI   **National Provider Identifier**
The NPI is a unique identification number for health care providers that will be used by all health plans. Health care providers and all health plans and health care clearinghouses will use the NPIs in the administrative and financial transactions specified by HIPAA. An NPI is a 10-position numeric identifier with a check digit in the last position to help detect keying errors. The NPI contains no embedded intelligence; that is, it contains no information about the health care provider such as the type of health care provider or State where the health care provider is located. (See NPPES)

NPPES   **National Plan and Provider Enumeration System**
The Administrative Simplification provisions of the Health Insurance Portability and Accountability Act of 1996 (HIPAA) mandated the adoption of standard unique identifiers for health care providers, as well as the adoption of standard unique identifiers for health plans. The purpose of these provisions is to improve the efficiency and effectiveness of the electronic transmission of health information. CMS has developed the NPPES to assign these unique identifiers.
https://nppes.cms.hhs.gov/NPPES/Welcome.do

NPRM **Notice of Proposed Rule Making**
A formal process through which government regulations (e.g., HIPAA standard transactions) are proposed for public comment before being adopted. Such NPRM's are published in the Federal Register and these notices discuss the legislative or other rationale for the proposed rule, and specify the length of the public comment period (e.g., 60 days). Comments received during this period are considered and responded to when the Final Rule is published.

NUBC **National Uniform Billing Committee**
The NUBC was brought together by the American Hospital Association (AHA) in 1975 and it includes the participation of all the major national provider and payer organizations. This committee was formed to develop a single billing form and standard data set that could be used nationwide by institutional providers and payers for handling health care claims.
www.nubc.org

NUCC **National Uniform Claim Committee**
The NUCC is a voluntary organization that replaced the Uniform Claim Form Task Force in 1995. This committee was created to develop a standardized data set for use by the non-institutional health care community to transmit claim and encounter information to and from all third-party payers. It is chaired by the American Medical Association (AMA), with the Centers for Medicare and Medicaid Services (CMS) as a critical partner. The committee includes representation from key provider and payer organizations, as well as standards setting organizations, state and federal regulators and the National Uniform Billing Committee (NUBC). The ADA's Dental Content Committee is an NUCC member organization.
www.nucc.org

OESS **Office of E-Health Standards and Services**
The office within CMS that develops and coordinates implementation of a comprehensive e-health strategy for CMS. Coordinates and supports internal and external technical activities related to e-health services (including parts of the Health Insurance Portability and Accountability Act (HIPAA)) and ensures that individual initiatives tie to the overall agency and Federal e-health goals and strategies.
www.cms.hhs.gov/CMSLeadership/14_Office_OESS.asp

OCR **Office for Civil Rights**
The Federal agency within HHS that is charged with enforcement of HIPAA privacy regulations.
www.hhs.gov/ocr/hipaa

POS   **Point of Service Plans**
A POS plan is a managed care program which allows subscribers to go to out of network providers. However, for this privilege, subscribers pay a higher premium and/or receive a lower reimbursement level.

PRO   **Peer Review Organizations**
Any group of medical professionals or a health care review company that includes licensed medical professionals approved by the state insurance department to analyze the quality and appropriateness of care rendered to patients. PROs were formerly known as professional standards review organizations.

QA   **Quality Assessment**
A methodology that obtains data that is used to evaluate the effectiveness of health care services and delivery. Surveys are one assessment tool. An objective of a quality assessment initiative is to determine what quality improvement actions may be appropriate.

QI / QIP   **Quality Improvement / Quality Improvement Program**
Programs whose central goal is to maintain what is good about the existing health care system while focusing on the areas that need improvement. A QIP is a set of related activities designed to achieve measurable improvement in processes and outcomes of care. Improvements are achieved through interventions that target health care providers, practitioners, plans, and/or beneficiaries.

RUC   **AMA / Relative Value System (RVS) Update Committee**
This committee supports maintenance of the CPT code set. Its role is to establish a standardized physician payment schedule based on a resource-based relative value scale (RBRVS). In the RBRVS system, payments for services are determined by the resource costs needed to provide them. The cost of providing each service is divided into three components: physician work, practice expense and professional liability insurance. Payments are calculated by multiplying the combined costs of a service by a conversion factor (a monetary amount that is determined by the Centers for Medicare and Medicaid Services). Payments are also adjusted for geographical differences in resource costs.
http://www.ama-assn.org/ama/pub/physician-resources/solutions-managing-your-practice/coding-billing-insurance/medicare/the-resource-based-relative-value-scale/the-rvs-update-committee.shtml

SCDI   **ADA Standards Committee on Dental Informatics**
The ADA develops standards for dental informatics through the SCDI, an ANSI accredited SDO. SCDI's mission is: "To promote patient care and oral health through the application of information technology to dentistry's clinical and administrative operations; to develop standards, specifications, technical reports, and guidelines for: components of a computerized dental clinical workstation; electronic technologies used in dental practice; and interoperability standards for different software and hardware products which provide a seamless information exchange throughout all facets of healthcare."

The SCDI is comprised of 60 voting members from 60 organizations (19 consumers, 21 producers, and 20 general interest) from the profession, dental industry, academia, and the government. In 2001, the SCDI was reorganized into four subcommittees and 14 working groups working on the development or revision of 26 technical reports or specifications. The actual standards development occurs in its 14 working groups. The subcommittees are grouped according to the following general subject matters: Dental Informatics Architecture and Devices, Electronic Dental Records, Informatic Component Interoperability in Dentistry, and Electronic Dissemination of Dental Information. The working groups, organized under the subcommittees, address specific topics and provide an opportunity for all interests to participate in the development of voluntary consensus standards. http://sitescape.ada.org/scdi (Note: This Web site requires special login and password access.)

SCHIP   **State Children's Health Insurance Program**
Dental services for the SCHIP are an optional benefit under Title XXI of the Social Security Act for all children up to age 19. However, nearly all States have opted to provide coverage for dental services. Under Title XXI, States have flexibility in targeting eligible uninsured children. States may choose to expand their Medicaid programs, design separate child health programs, or create a combination of both.

SDO   **Standards Development Organization**
A term used in HIPAA regulations that denotes ANSI ASC's whose mission includes developing the technical solution for transmitting health care information through standard electronic transactions. There are three SDOs identified under HIPAA, Health Level 7, X12 and the National Council for Prescription Drug Programs.

SNODENT **Systematized Nomenclature of Dentistry**
SNODENT is a large codified taxonomy of dentally related terms and descriptors that can be used to fully describe a patient's condition and dental diagnosis in an electronic medium. The development of dental diagnostic codes was initially recommended by action of the House of Delegates in Resolution 74H-1990 (Trans.1990:542). This taxonomy was based on the SNOMED architecture under an agreement between the ADA and CAP. (See SNOMED)

SNOMED/ **Systematized Nomenclature of Medicine – Clinical Terms**
SNOMED CT SNOMED / SNOMED CT is a scientifically validated clinical health care terminology and infrastructure that makes health care knowledge more usable and accessible. The SNOMED CT Core terminology provides a common language that enables a consistent way of capturing, sharing and aggregating health data across specialties and sites of care. Among the applications for SNOMED CT are electronic medical records, ICU monitoring, clinical decision support, medical research studies, clinical trials, computerized physician order entry, disease surveillance, image indexing and consumer health information services.
www.ihtsdo.org

TDP/TFD **TRICARE Dental Program / TRICARE Family Dental Program**
The TRICARE Dental Program (TDP) is offered by the Department of Defense (DoD) through the TRICARE Management Activity (TMA). United Concordia Companies, Inc. administers and underwrites the TDP for the TMA. The TDP is a high-quality, cost-effective dental care benefit for eligible family members of all active duty uniformed services personnel; as well members of the Selected Reserve and Individual Ready Reserve (IRR) and their eligible family members.
http:/www.tricare.mil/mybenefit/home/Dental

TPA **Third-Party Administrator**
Claims payer who assumes responsibility for administering health benefit plans without assuming any financial risk. Some commercial insurance carriers and Blue Cross/Blue Shield plans also have TPA operations to accommodate self-funded employers seeking administrative services only (ASO) contracts.

TR3 **Technical Report 3 (replacement term for: IG/Implementation Guide)**

TRICARE **Acronym for CHAMPUS' replacement program.**
http://www.tricare.mil

UR	**Utilization Review**
	A program for determining what health care services are covered and payable under the health plan and the extent of such coverage and payments. Such reviews come before the service (pre-determination) or after the fact (retrospective).

WEDI	**Workgroup for Electronic Data Interchange**
	WEDI's "CORE PURPOSE" is to improve the quality of healthcare through effective and efficient information exchange and management. Its MISSION is to provide leadership and guidance to the healthcare industry on how to use and leverage the industry's collective knowledge, expertise and information resources to improve the quality, affordability and availability of healthcare.
	www.wedi.org

WEDI SNIP	**Workgroup for Electronic Data Interchange – Strategic National Implementation Process**
	SNIP is a collaborative healthcare industry-wide process resulting in the implementation of standards and furthering the development and implementation of future standards. WEDI SNIP has been established to meet the immediate need to assess industry-wide HIPAA Administrative Simplification implementation readiness and to bring about the national coordination necessary for successful compliance.
	http://www.wedi.org/snip/

WHO	**World Health Organization**
	WHO is the United Nations specialized agency for health. It was established on 7 April 1948. The agency's objective, as set out in its Constitution, is the attainment by all peoples of the highest possible level of health. Health is defined in WHO's Constitution as a state of complete physical, mental and social well-being and not merely the absence of disease or infirmity.
	http://www.who.int/en

X12/X12N	**See ANSI ASC X12N**
	www.X12.org (from the "Committees/Groups" drop-down menu select Subcommittees then Insurance)

Numeric Index to Procedure Codes in CDT Companion

13

CDT
Companion

ADA American Dental Association®
America's leading advocate for oral health

Chapter 13
Numeric Index to Procedure Codes in CDT Companion

From the *Code on Dental Procedures and Nomenclature (Code)*

I. Diagnostic

Procedure Code	Page References by CDT Companion Section	
	Coding Exercises (Chapter 5)	Cross Coding (Chapter 9)
D0120	38, 39, 41, 58	–
D0140	47, 71, 79, 82	219
D0145	41, 113	–
D0150	38, 57, 58, 70, 85	220
D0160	71	221
D0170	–	222
D0180	58, 85	–
D0210	42	223
D0220	43, 82, 85	223
D0230	43, 82, 85	224
D0273	85	–
D0274	43	–
D0320	–	224
D0321	–	225
D0330	43	225
D0340	57	226
D0350	57	–
D0360	61	–
D0362	61, 63	–
D0363	61	–
D0431	59	–
D0460	56	–
D0470	57	–
D0999	59	–

II. Preventive

Procedure Code	Page References by CDT Companion Section	
	Coding Exercises (Chapter 5)	Cross Coding (Chapter 9)
D1110	39, 44, 90, 100, 101	–
D1120	38, 41	–
D1203	38, 41	–
D1204	37, 39	–
D1206	37, 41, 51	–
D1320	87	–
D1351	51, 102	–
D1352	103	–
D1555	38, 39	–

III. Restorative

Procedure Code	Page References by CDT Companion Section	
	Coding Exercises (Chapter 5)	Cross Coding (Chapter 9)
D2391	51, 102	–
D2392	51	–
D2393	51	–
D2740	49	–
D2752	47	–
D2790	65	–
D2934	81	–
D2950	47	–
D2952	45, 49	–
D2954	45	–
D2970	47	–
D2971	65	–
D2999	51, 98	–

IV. Endodontics

	Page References by CDT Companion Section	
Procedure Code	Coding Exercises (Chapter 5)	Cross Coding (Chapter 9)
D3221	95, 97	–
D3222	56	–
D3230	81	–
D3320	56, 95, 97	–
D3330	56	–
D3332	97	–
D3410	–	227
D3421	–	227
D3425	–	227
D3426	–	227
D3430	–	228
D3450	–	228
D3470	–	229

V. Periodontics

Procedure Code	Page References by CDT Companion Section	
	Coding Exercises (Chapter 5)	Cross Coding (Chapter 9)
D4210	–	231
D4211	93	231
D4230	–	232
D4231	–	232
D4240	–	232
D4241	83, 89	232
D4245	–	233
D4249	–	233
D4260	89	234
D4261	–	234
D4263	89, 107	–
D4266	89	235
D4267	–	235
D4270	–	236
D4271	–	236
D4273	–	236
D4275	–	236
D4276	–	236
D4342	75, 83, 87, 90	–
D4355	85	–
D4381	87	–
D4999	83, 87	–

VI. Prosthodontics, removable

Procedure Code	Page References by CDT Companion Section	
	Coding Exercises (Chapter 5)	Cross Coding (Chapter 9)
D5650	65	–
D5660	65	–

VII. Maxillofacial Prosthetics

Procedure Code	Page References by CDT Companion Section	
	Coding Exercises (Chapter 5)	Cross Coding (Chapter 9)
D5931	–	237
D5932	–	237
D5936	–	237
D5999	53	238

VIII. Implant Services

Procedure Code	Page References by CDT Companion Section	
	Coding Exercises (Chapter 5)	Cross Coding (Chapter 9)
D6010	67	239
D6012	63	239
D6040	–	239
D6050	–	239
D6053	–	–
D6055	67	–
D6056	67	–
D6100	–	240
D6190	–	241

IX. Prosthodontics, fixed

Procedure Code	Page References by CDT Companion Section	
	Coding Exercises (Chapter 5)	Cross Coding (Chapter 9)
D6242	69	–
D6545	69	–
D6548	69	–
D6970	45	–
D6972	45	–
D6999	69	–

X. Oral and Maxillofacial Surgery

	Page References by CDT Companion Section	
Procedure Code	Coding Exercises (Chapter 5)	Cross Coding (Chapter 9)
D7140	65, 72, 75	–
D7210	65	243
D7220	–	243
D7230	–	243
D7240	–	243
D7241	–	243
D7250	–	244
D7251	105	–
D7260	–	244
D7270	–	245
D7285	–	245
D7286	91	246
D7287	91	–
D7288	85, 91	247
D7292	63	–
D7293	61, 63	–
D7294	61, 63	–
D7295	107	–
D7310	–	248
D7311	–	248
D7320	–	248
D7321	–	248
D7340	–	249
D7350	–	249
D7410	–	250
D7411	–	250
D7412	–	250
D7413	–	251
D7414	–	251
D7415	–	251
D7440	–	252
D7441	–	252
D7465	–	253
D7471	–	253
D7472	–	253

X. Oral and Maxillofacial Surgery (continued)

	Page References by CDT Companion Section	
Procedure Code	Coding Exercises (Chapter 5)	Cross Coding (Chapter 9)
D7473	–	253
D7485	–	254
D7490	–	254
D7510	83	255
D7511	–	255
D7520	–	256
D7521	–	256
D7530	–	257
D7540	–	257
D7550	–	258
D7560	–	258
D7610	–	259
D7620	–	259
D7630	–	259
D7640	–	259
D7650	–	260
D7660	–	260
D7670	–	260
D7671	–	260
D7680	–	261
D7710	–	261
D7720	–	262
D7730	–	261
D7740	–	262
D7750	–	262
D7760	–	262
D7770	–	263
D7771	–	263
D7780	–	263
D7810	–	264
D7820	–	264
D7830	–	264
D7840	–	265
D7850	–	265
D7852	–	266

X. Oral and Maxillofacial Surgery (continued)

Procedure Code	Page References by CDT Companion Section	
	Coding Exercises (Chapter 5)	Cross Coding (Chapter 9)
D7854	–	266
D7856	–	267
D7858	–	267
D7860	–	268
D7865	–	268
D7870	–	269
D7871	–	269
D7872	–	270
D7873	–	270
D7874	–	270
D7875	–	270
D7876	–	270
D7877	–	270
D7880	71	271
D7899	73	–
D7910	77	271
D7911	–	272
D7912	–	272
D7920	–	273
D7940	–	273
D7941	–	274
D7943	–	274
D7944	–	274
D7945	–	275
D7946	–	276
D7947	–	277
D7948	–	277
D7949	–	278
D7950	–	279
D7951	–	279
D7953	107	280
D7955	107	280
D7960	–	281
D7963	–	281
D7970	–	281

X. Oral and Maxillofacial Surgery (continued)

| Procedure Code | Page References by CDT Companion Section | |
	Coding Exercises (Chapter 5)	Cross Coding (Chapter 9)
D7971	–	282
D7972	–	282
D7980	–	283
D7981	–	283
D7982	–	284
D7983	–	284
D7990	–	285
D7991	–	285
D7995	–	286
D7996	–	286
D7997	–	287
D7998	–	287

XI. Adjunctive General Services

| Procedure Code | Page References by CDT Companion Section | |
	Coding Exercises (Chapter 5)	Cross Coding (Chapter 9)
D9120	75	–
D9212	–	289
D9215	87	–
D9220	–	289
D9221	–	289
D9230	77	–
D9241	–	290
D9242	–	290
D9248	77	–
D9310	79, 105	291
D9440	47	–
D9450	57	–
D9610	77	–
D9630	85	–
D9910	37	–
D9920	81	–
D9941	77	–

From the Current Procedure Terminology (CPT)

Procedure Code	Page References by CDT Companion Section	
	Coding Exercises (Chapter 5)	Cross Coding (Chapter 9)
10061	–	256
11100	–	246
11101	–	246
11641	–	251
12053	–	272
13152	–	272
20000	–	255
20240	–	245
20245	–	245
20520	–	257
20605	–	269
20670	–	240, 287
20680	–	240, 287
20694	–	287
20900	–	279, 280
20902	–	279
21010	–	268
21031	–	253
21032	–	253
21044	–	252
21045	–	254
21050	–	265
21060	–	265
21070	–	285
21125	–	279
21141	–	276
21145	–	276
21150	–	277
21154	–	278
21193	–	274
21194	–	274
21198	–	274, 275
21206	–	274
21240	–	268
21248	–	239

From the Current Procedure Terminology (CPT) (continued)

Procedure Code	Page References by CDT Companion Section	
	Coding Exercises (Chapter 5)	Cross Coding (Chapter 9)
21249	–	239
21360	–	260, 262
21421	–	262
21422	–	261
21432	–	259
21440	–	259, 260, 263
21445	–	260, 263
21450	–	259, 262
21462	–	259
21465	–	261
21480	–	264
21485	–	264
21490	–	264
21497	–	261, 263, 287
29800	–	270
29804	–	270
30580	–	244
31030	–	244
31603	–	285
31605	–	285
40702	–	280
40799	–	247
40804	–	257
40810	–	250, 251
40812	–	250, 251
40814	–	250, 251
40831	–	271
40842	–	249
40843	–	249
40844	–	249
40899	–	247
41010	–	281
41015	–	255, 256
41115	–	281
41252	–	272

From the Current Procedure Terminology (CPT) (continued)

Procedure Code	Page References by CDT Companion Section	
	Coding Exercises (Chapter 5)	Cross Coding (Chapter 9)
41520	–	281
41599	–	247
41805	–	257
41806	–	257
41820	–	231
41821	–	282
41822	–	282
41823	–	254
41828	–	281
41830	–	258
41870	–	236
41872	–	231
41874	–	248
41899	–	227, 228, 229, 232, 233, 234, 235, 241, 243, 244, 245, 269, 271
42330	–	283
42335	–	283
42440	–	283
42450	–	283
42500	–	284
42505	–	284
42600	–	284
64400	–	289
70300	–	223
70310	–	224
70320	–	223
70328	–	225
70330	–	225
70332	–	224
70350	–	226
70355	–	225
99201	–	219
99212	–	219, 222

From the Current Procedure Terminology (CPT) (continued)

Procedure Code	Page References by CDT Companion Section	
	Coding Exercises (Chapter 5)	Cross Coding (Chapter 9)
99213	–	221, 222
99214	–	221
99215	–	220
99241	–	291
99242	–	291

From the Healthcare Common Procedure Coding System (HCPCS)

Procedure Code	Page References by CDT Companion Section	
	Coding Exercises (Chapter 5)	Cross Coding (Chapter 9)
E0485	–	238
E0486	53	238
S8262	71	271

Alphabetic Index – Coding Exercises/Quizzes/Sidebars

14

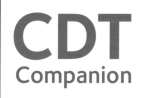

Chapter 14 - Alphabetic Index – Coding Exercises/Quizzes/Sidebars

Subject / Term	Chapter 5 Page References			
	Exercise		Quiz/Sidebar	
	#	Page	#	Page
Abscess	19	83	-	-
Additional procedures to construct crown	12	65	-	-
Addition of clasp to partial denture	12	65	-	-
Age of Child	2	39	-	-
Analgesia, anxiolysis, nitrous oxide	17	77	-	-
Apexogenesis	-	-	3b	56
Appliance	15	71	6	73
Area of the oral cavity on claims	-	-	7a, 10	78, 99
Athletic mouthguard	17	77	-	-
Atridox®/Arrestin®/Actisite®/Periochip®	20 (part 2)	87	-	-
Behavior management	18	81	-	-
Biopsy				
Brush	20 (part 1)	85	Sidebar	91
Cytology sample collection	20 (part 1)	85	Sidebar	91
Soft tissue		-	Sidebar	91
Bone				
harvest of	27	107	-	-
replacement graft	20 (part 3)	89	-	-
Buccal pit restoration	7	50	-	-
CAD/CAM	6	49	-	-
Cancer screening	10	58	-	-
Case presentation	-	-	4a	57
Chemiluminescent testing	10	59	-	-
Chlorhexidine gluconate rinse	19, 20 (parts 1-2)	82, 84, 85, 86	-	-
Clear Aligners	-	-	4b	57
Cone beam ct			Sidebar	62
Cephalometric view	-	-	5b	63
Data capture	11	61	Sidebar	62
2-dimensional reconstruction	11	61	Sidebar 5b	63 63
3-dimensional reconstruction	11	61	Sidebar	62
Connecting bar	13	67	-	-

Subject / Term	Chapter 5 Page References			
	Exercise		Quiz/Sidebar	
	#	Page	#	Page
Consultation	26	105	8a, b	79
Conservative Resin Restoration (See Preventive Resin Restoration)	25	103		
Coronectomy	26	105	–	–
Core buildup	5	47	–	–
Crown				
All ceramic	6	49	–	–
Primary tooth	18	81	–	–
PFM (porcelain fused to metal)	5, 14	46, 69	–	–
Porcelain/ceramic	6, 14	49, 69	–	–
Temporary crown	5	47	–	–
Prefabricated stainless steel	18	81	–	–
To fit partial denture	12	65	–	–
Curettage	19	82	Sidebar	91
Date of service	–	–	9	90
Endodontic treatment	9	54	3a	56
Prosthodontic treatment	9	54	–	–
Debridement (full mouth)	20 (part 1)	85	–	–
Desensitizing medicament (application of)	1	37	–	–
Diagnostic casts	–	–	4a	57
Diet	3	40	–	–
Downcoding	2, 4	39, 43	–	–
Drugs and medicaments	20 (part 1)	85	–	–
Extraction – erupted tooth or exposed root	12, 15, 16	65, 72, 75	–	–
Endodontic therapy	22, 23	95, 97	3a	56
Endosteal implant placement	13	67	–	–
ERA attachment	13	66	–	–
Fixed partial denture				
Retainers	14	69	2	45
Sectioning	16	74, 75	–	–
Fractured root	23	97	–	–
Fluoride				
Varnish	1, 3, 7	36, 40, 50	–	–
Topical application	1, 2, 3	37, 41	–	–
Full mouth series	4, 20 (part 1)	42, 85	–	–
Gingival flap procedure	19, 20 (part 3)	83, 89	–	–

Subject / Term	Chapter 5 Page References			
	Exercise		Quiz/Sidebar	
	#	Page	#	Page
Gingivectomy or gingivoplasty	21	93	–	–
Guided tissue regeneration	20 (part 3)	89	–	–
Hadar bar	13	66	–	–
Harvesting bone	27	106	–	–
Incision and drainage of abscess	19	83	–	–
Implant abutment	13	67	–	–
Implant/abutment supported removable denture	13	67	–	–
Intra-oral staining technique	10	59	–	–
Invisalign (see Clear Alingers)	–	–	4b	57
Local Anesthesia	20 (part 2)	87	–	–
Localized delivery of antimicrobial agents	20 (part 2)	87	–	–
Maryland bridge	14	68	–	–
Mouthguard	17	77	–	–
New patient	2	38	4a	57
Non-intravenous conscious sedation	17	77	–	–
Occlusal orthotic device	15	71	–	–
Office visit – after hours	5	47	–	–
Osseous surgery	20 (part 3)	88, 89	–	–
Oral Evaluation				
Comprehensive	2, 10, 15, 20 (part 1)	38, 58, 70, 85	4a	57
Comprehensive periodontal	20 (part 1)	85	–	–
Limited	5, 15, 19	47, 71, 82, 83	8b	79
Patient under 3	3	41	–	–
Periodic	2, 10	38, 58	–	–
Problem focused	15	71	–	–
Palliative	19	82	–	–
Periodontal maintenance	20 (part 3), 24	88, 100, 101	–	–
Periodontal scaling and root planing	16, 19, 20 (part 2)	75, 83, 87	9	90
Pontic – porcelain fused to metal	14	69	–	–
Post and core				
Indirectly fabricated	6	49	2	45
Prefabricated	–	–	2	45

Subject / Term	Chapter 5 Page References			
	Exercise		Quiz/Sidebar	
	#	Page	#	Page
Preventive resin restoration	25	102, 103	–	–
Prophylaxis (child / adult)	2, 3	38, 39, 41	1, 9	44, 90
Partial	–	–	1	44
On recall after periodontal therapy	24	100	–	–
Pulp vitality test	–	–	3a	56
Pulpal debridement	22, 23	95, 97	–	
Pulpal therapy	18	81	–	–
Radiographs/Images				
Full mouth series	4, 20 (part 1)	42, 85	–	–
Panoramic film	4	42, 43	–	–
Periapical film	4, 19, 20 (part 1)	42, 43, 82 84, 85	Sidebar	62
Bitewing film	4, 20 (part 1)	42, 43, 84, 85	–	–
Cephalometric film	–	–	4a, 5b Sidebar	57, 63 62
Oral/facial photographic	–	–	4a	57
Restoration		–	–	
preventive resin	25	102, 103		
resin based composite	7	51	–	–
Root canal	9, 22, 23	54, 55, 94, 95, 96, 97	3b	56
Root tip removal	12	65	–	–
Sealant	2, 25	39, 51, 102	–	–
Section fixed partial denture	16	74, 75	–	–
Sextants	–	–	10	99
Site	20 (part 3)	89	–	–
Sleep apnea device	8	53	–	–
Suture of small wound	17	77	–	–
Therapeutic drug injection	17	77	–	–
Temporary implant				
Placement	11	60, 61	–	–
Removal	–	–	5a	63
TMJ (temporomandibular joint)	15	70, 71	6	73
Tobacco counseling	20 (part 2)	87	–	–
Toluidine blue	10	59	–	–

Subject / Term	Chapter 5 Page References			
	Exercise		Quiz/Sidebar	
	#	Page	#	Page
Tooth brush deplaquing	3	40	–	–
Tooth numbers on claims	21	93	7b	78
Unspecified procedure, by report			Sidebar	98
Diagnostic	10	59	–	–
Maxillofacial Prosthetics	8	53	–	–
Oral & Maxillofacial Surgery	17	77	–	–
Periodontal	19	83	–	–
Prosthodontic	14	69	–	–
Restorative	7	51	Sidebar	98
TMD therapy	–	–	6	73
Vizilite®	10	59	–	–
Widman surgery	20 (part 3)	88	–	–